LOW FODMAP DIET COOKBOOK

Essential Guide of Low Fodmap Diet Plus Simple Recipes

(Improve Digestion, With Easy, Healthy and Satisfying Recipes)

Amber Crain

Published by Alex Howard

© **Amber Crain**

All Rights Reserved

Low Fodmap Diet Cookbook: Essential Guide of Low Fodmap Diet Plus Simple Recipes (Improve Digestion, With Easy, Healthy and Satisfying Recipes)

ISBN 978-1-990169-22-9

All rights reserved. No part of this guide may be reproduced in any form without permission in writing from the publisher except in the case of brief quotations embodied in critical articles or reviews.

Legal & Disclaimer

The information contained in this book is not designed to replace or take the place of any form of medicine or professional medical advice. The information in this book has been provided for educational and entertainment purposes only.

The information contained in this book has been compiled from sources deemed reliable, and it is accurate to the best of the Author's knowledge; however, the Author cannot guarantee its accuracy and validity and cannot be held liable for any errors or omissions. Changes are periodically made to this book. You must consult your doctor or get professional medical advice before using any of the suggested remedies, techniques, or information in this book.

Table of contents

PART 1 1

INTRODUCTION 2

Bircher Muesli (Serves 1) 10
Orange And Ginger Compote 12
Carrot And Orange Breakfast Bars (Makes 12) 14
Baked Ham And Eggs (Serves 1-2) 16
Low Fodmap Omelette (Serves 1) 18
Butternut Squash And Mixed Spice Muffins (Makes 12) 20
Kedgeree (Serves 2) 22
Shakshuka (Serves 2-4) 24
Quinoa Porridge (Serves 1) 26
Breakfast Burgers (Makes 2) 28
Breakfast Chimichangas (Serves 1) 30

SOUPS 31

Tomato And Carrot Soup (Serves 2) 32
Curried Coconut And Parsnip (Serves 4-6) 34
Winter Vegetable Broth (Serves 4) 35
Carrot And Coconut Soup (Serves 2) 37
Minestrone (Serves 4) 39
Cream Of Mushroom Soup (Serves 2) 41
Chicken Soup (Serves 4) 43
Fish Chowder (Serves 2-4) 45
Potato And Chive Soup (Serves 4) 47
Butternut Squash And Ginger (Serves 4) 49

LIGHT MEALS, LUNCHES AND SNACKS 51

Roasted New Potato Salad (Serves 1) 52
Taquitos (Serves 4) 54
Caprese Bruschetta (Serves 2) 56
Halloumi Fries (Serves 2) 58
Chicken Burritos (Serves 4) 60
Gluten-Free Pizzas (Serves 1) 62

Dirty Fries (Serves 2-4) 64
Popcorn Chicken (Serves 2-4) 66
Cornish Pasties (Makes 6) 68
Spiced Sweet Potato And Feta Wraps (Serves 4) 70
Vegetable Samosas (Makes 8) 72
Roasted Red Pepper And Tomato Salad (Serves 4) 74

SIDES 75

Ratatouille (Serves 4-6) 76
Baba Ganoush (Serves 6) 78
Roasted Carrot Hummus (Serves 6) 80
Blue Cheese Salad Dressing (Serves 4) 82
Basil And Pine Nut Pesto (Serves 5) 84
Onion And Garlic Infused Oils 86
Stuffed Potato Skins (Serves 2-4) 88
Sesame Sautéed Broccoli And Red Pepper (Serves 2) 90
Greek Salad (Serves 1 As A Main Or 2 As A Side) 92
Roasted Radishes (Serves 4) 94
Crispy Kale (Serves 2) 96
Cheese And Chive Baked Baguettes (Serves 2-4) 97
Sage And 'Onion' Stuffing (Serves 4-8) 99
Spiced Red Cabbage (Serves 10-14) 101

PART 2 103

INTRODUCTION 104

WHAT ARE FODMAPS 105

The Different Fodmaps 107

OVERVIEW OF FODMAP-POOR AND FODMAP-RICH FOODS 109

How Do Fodmaps Cause Symptoms Of Ibs? 110
Why Don't We All Suffer From Pds? 112
To Investigate 113
Intestinal Complaints 114

FOLLOW THE FODMAP DIET 115

LOW-FODMAP DIET DURING THE FESTIVE PERIODS. 117

THE 3 DIET PHASES: **120**

Low And High Fodmap Products 121

HIGH FODMAP PRODUCTS **121**

HERE ARE EXAMPLES OF FODMAP RECIPES **136**

Lettuce Tacos With Chicken To The Shepherd 136
Apple Salad With Garbanzo And Nut 139
Sheet Pan Steak Fajitas 141
Sheet Pan Tuscan Chicken 143
Breaded Pork Chop Sheet Pan Dinner 146
Eggplant Stuffed With Tomato With Tzatziki 149
Vegetable And Kale Soup 151
Salad With Fried Goat Cheese 153
Steamed Cod 155
Vegetable Lasagna 157
Lemon-Garlic-Zucchini Salad With Walnuts And Ricotta Cheese 159
Tuna And Vegetable Salad 161
Potato And Vegetable Salad With Herb Dressing 162
Salad With Asparagus, Cherry Tomatoes, And Cottage Cheese 164
Oven Dish With Creamy Brussels Sprouts 166
Poké Bowl With Salmon 168
Burritos Of Cabbage 170
Waffle With Sausage Cheese Flour 172
Oopsie Bread 173
Leek Minced Almond Flour Pastry 174
Thai Pumpkin Soup 176
Colorful Asparagus Caprese Salad 178
Bowl Of Shawarma 180
Blue Corded Chicken Breast 182
Duck Breast With Mirabelle Plums 184
Steamed Cod 186
Soup With Rice, Potatoes And Chicken 188

CONCLUSION **189**

Part 1

Introduction

I really enjoy cooking low FODMAP food and trying new FODMAP friendly recipes, but I frequently hear readers say that they won't try to cook low FODMAP recipes themselves because it seems too hard and that they don't feel that they have the skills to create a dish from scratch, a belief which is often wrong. Most FODMAP friendly home cooking isn't hard and can be considerably healthier than a shop-bought version, so the mission statement of The Fat Foodie is to help make cooking low FODMAP food easy, relatively fast, and uncomplicated. In other words, I'm committed to making low FODMAP food good!

Once I had educated myself as to how the low FODMAP diet worked I was astonished at how much of the food I'd been eating previously had been high FODMAP. Aside from eating onion and garlic on a daily basis I'd also been eating high FODMAP foods, such as beans, chickpeas, cauliflower, apples, pears, cheese, pasta, noodles and gluten-based foods, very regularly. It was no wonder I'd been in such discomfort.

Another aspect of my low FODMAP education which massively opened my eyes was discovering the extent to which pre-packaged foods (in every form) were unsuitable on a low FODMAP diet. So many of them contained onion or garlic as flavourings and seasonings and were trigger foods as a result. Accordingly, this made me realise the importance of being able to cook my own low FODMAP food, so I began to develop family-friendly low FODMAP recipes that wouldn't cause me to have digestive problems, but were tasty enough for my whole family to enjoy.

At the time of writing this cookbook there are very few companies in Britain who make and supply low FODMAP foods, either as dry pantry ingredients, chilled pre-prepared foods or in frozen form. For this reason it makes sense to cook your own food when you can because it gives you the power to control the quantity of FODMAPs you're ingesting, rather than buying pre-prepared foods that could have hidden high FODMAPs in them disguised as seasonings or flavourings.

The FODMAP Diet:

Irritable Bowel Syndrome (IBS) is a medical term which refers to a common condition which affects the digestive system, causing symptoms which include stomach cramps, diarrhoea, constipation, bloating, flatulence, tiredness, nausea, heartburn, indigestion and even urinary issues. According to the IBS Network, between 10 and 20% of the British population at any one time is suffering from IBS[1], while Monash University states that 15% of the population worldwide (1 in 7 people) suffer from IBS.[2] These statistics demonstrate that it is a condition which affects a huge proportion of people. There is no known specific cause for IBS, but following a low FODMAP diet can successfully manage the symptoms for approximately 75-80% of people who suffer from IBS.

The low FODMAP diet was discovered and developed in 1999 by a team at Monash University in Australia. Their research showed that there are a specific collection of carbohydrates, which they called FODMAPs, which cause discomfort to IBS sufferers because their bodies struggle to absorb and process them correctly within the small intestine. As a result, the undigested carbohydrates are fermented inside the large intestine, which causes fluid absorption and fermentation and therefore, IBS symptoms and discomfort.

These FODMAPs are:

Fermentable: (In which the bacteria in the gut ferments undigested carbohydrates which in turn creates gas and therefore, flatulence)

Oligosaccharides: (which include Fructo-oligosaccharides (FOS) which are found in wheat, rye, onions and garlic and Galacto-oligosaccharides (GOS) which are found in legumes/beans and pulses)

Disaccharides: (Lactose which is naturally found in dairy foods, such as milk, soft cheese and yoghurt)

Mono-saccharide: (Fructose, a carbohydrate found in honey, apples, as well as high fructose corn syrups etc.)

and Polyols: (Sugar polyols, such as sorbitol and mannitol, which are found in particular fruits and vegetables and can also be used in artificial sweeteners).

In essence, the low FODMAP diet works by limiting foods which are high in FODMAPs, thereby lowering the frequency of IBS attacks in patients. As a result, 75-80% of IBS sufferers report that following the low FODMAP diet enables them to control their symptoms.

Following the FODMAP diet:

The low FODMAP diet has three distinct phases. The first is the elimination or restriction phase in which all high FODMAP foods are removed from the diet for a period of 2 to 6 weeks and only low FODMAP foods are eaten in FODMAP-safe portion sizes. This is to essentially wipe the slate clean of FODMAP triggers in order to help identify problematic foods in the second stage. The first stage should only be used for 2 to 6 weeks in order to ensure that long-term gut health is not affected.

The second stage is re-challenge and re-introduction in which your individual tolerance levels to each of the high FODMAP groups are tested. In this stage, in one week a specific FODMAP group is challenged on 2 to 3 days and your gut's response to that particular group is monitored over the course of the week in order to determine your individual toleration levels.

The last stage is simply living on your own adapted low FODMAP diet.

Although I began the low FODMAP diet on my own it is strongly advised that you speak to your doctor before self-diagnosing IBS because there are many conditions which can be confused with IBS and it is very important to rule them out. These conditions can include coeliac/celiac disease, Crohn's disease, inflammatory bowel disease, cancer etc. Also, even if you are diagnosed with IBS it is advised that you proceed with the low FODMAP diet under the instruction of a registered dietician or nutritionist because it is important to ensure that your body is receiving the correct dietary requirements while eliminating problematic high FODMAP-containing foods from your diet.

I do acknowledge however, that the NHS is under a great amount of strain and it is not always possible to receive a referral to see a specialist, or certainly not in a timely fashion, in which case I would recommend that you purchase the Monash University FODMAP app and follow the guidance it provides. There is also an extensive list of resources at the back of this book.

Disclaimer: As with any medical issue, it is important that you speak to your doctor or health professional before self-diagnosing yourself with IBS because there are a number of health conditions which have symptoms that mirror that of IBS. Therefore, it's best to consult your doctor to rule out any illnesses which are more serious than IBS. Also, this book and my website are not intended to be used as a full guide to the low FODMAP diet, it is simply my way of sharing low FODMAP recipes with other FODMAP diet followers who have received a diagnosis of IBS. If you think you would benefit from following the low FODMAP diet you should first speak to a doctor or registered dietitian.

About the low FODMAP recipes in this book:

The recipes in this book were created following the recommended low FODMAP levels of Monash University's app, so they are all officially low FODMAP. However, I must stress once again that I am not a dietitian or nutritionist and I cannot understate the importance of consulting your GP or a registered dietitian or nutritionist before commencing the low FODMAP diet.

These recipes are, quite simply, what I eat. They were created to ensure that I didn't have to cook separate meals for myself and so my family could enjoy exactly the same meals as me. In a way, that was the ultimate test: to make low FODMAP food good. If a recipe states that it 'serves 4' or 'makes 4' that means that 1 serving or piece is a low FODMAP portion unless otherwise stated within the text of the recipe.

When I began the low FODMAP diet I couldn't envision being able to make tasty food that didn't contain onions, garlic, dairy, beans and the likes, but it **is** possible and it can be done well. There is no need to miss out on flavour just because you're omitting the higher FODMAP foods.

These recipes are highly adaptable and can easily be made dairy-free, gluten-free, vegetarian and vegan. It's relatively easy nowadays to find non-dairy and gluten-free versions of foods and the range is growing on a daily basis. Here are a few ingredient options which you can utilise to make your food more FODMAP friendly:

Milk alternatives:

I use rice milk because I have a low level allergy to dairy and I find rice milk to be the most useful of the milk alternatives on the market. It does not have a strong taste, it's got a creamy feel to it and it doesn't curdle in hot liquids like many other options do. It's also low FODMAP at a serving of 200ml. However, there are other milk alternatives which can be used, such as almond milk (low FODMAP up to 250ml per serving), UHT coconut milk (low FODMAP up to 125ml per serving), hemp milk (low FODMAP up to 250ml per serving) and macadamia milk (low FODMAP up to 250ml per serving). Soy milk tends to be problematic due to its production method, so I'd advise giving it a miss.

It is important to stress though, that the low FODMAP diet isn't necessarily a dairy-free one because it is only the carbohydrate lactose which is the issue at hand therefore, lactose-free products can safely be eaten on the low FODMAP diet, assuming you're not allergic to dairy.

Gluten-free products:

When the low FODMAP diet began it was believed that gluten itself was the problem when it came to causing digestive problems. However, it has recently been discovered that, unless you are coeliac, it is not gluten which causes the issue, it's the fructan carbohydrates found in wheat. As a result, wheat flour which has been processed further to wash away these fructans has been found to be low FODMAP.

Sadly, at present this flour is only available in Australian shops at the moment, but you can buy it online in Britain. However, there are a multitude of gluten-free flours available in Britain and many of them can be used in low FODMAP recipes without affecting the taste. These flours can include: almond flour (low FODMAP up to 24g per serving), arrowroot, buckwheat (low FODMAP up to 100g per serving), cornflour (low FODMAP up to 100g per serving), green banana (low FODMAP up to 100g per serving), maize (low FODMAP up to 100g per serving), maize starch (low FODMAP up to 100g per serving), millet (low FODMAP up to 100g per serving), quinoa (low FODMAP up to 100g per serving), rice (low FODMAP up to 100g per serving), sorghum (low FODMAP up to 100g per serving), teff (low FODMAP up to 100g per serving), yam (low FODMAP up to 100g per serving), potato starch (low FODMAP up to 100g per serving) and tapioca starch (low FODMAP up to 100g per serving).

Flours to avoid due to their high FODMAP levels are rye, amaranth, soy, barley, coconut, einkorn, emmer, Khorasan (kamut), lupin, spelt and wheat.

Spelt flour is unique in that on its own it is a high FODMAP flour, but if it is used to bake traditional spelt sourdough bread the fermentation process breaks down the FODMAPs and tends to make it low in FODMAPs. However, each sourdough recipe would have its own FODMAP content which would need to be considered on an individual basis.

Another aspect of gluten-free bread to consider is whether it has any high FODMAP ingredients added to it, such as inulin. Although you can make your own gluten-free flour blend at home, I think the easiest way is to find a ready-made gluten-free flour blend which has no high FODMAP ingredients in it and use it. As far as I'm concerned, life's too short to be measuring out my own flour blend! (I use **DOVE'S FARM**.)

Although I always use gluten-free flour because it prevents me from having digestive discomfort it can be a bit more difficult to work with than normal wheat flour. It often requires more liquid in the recipes it's used in because of the absorbent nature of the ingredients it's made from and the finished product tends to be crumblier than those made with wheat flour due to the lack of gluten. This can be resolved by using xanthan gum or guar gum because they emulsify, thicken and stabilise gluten-free flours, helping to improve the overall texture. Although both of these products are low FODMAP they can sometimes cause gas and bloating for some people, so you would need to test your own body's response to them.

Other considerations on the low FODMAP diet:

There are other things to consider when eating on the low FODMAP diet, such as limiting the amount of fat you consume. Although fats are not high FODMAP, too much fat in the diet can increase gut motility. In other words, it can make you poo more and have looser bowel movements or experience constipation. Alcohol is a gut irritant too, as is caffeine and carbonated drinks. Spicy food can cause issues for IBS sufferers because although chillies are low FODMAP (in no more than a 28g serving) they contain a substance called capsaicin which produces the spiciness of chillies and can sometimes irritate the gut.

Resistant starches can also be problematic for those with IBS. Resistant starch is formed in starch-containing foods when they have been cooked and cooled down, particularly if they are then reheated, such as in the case of potatoes, legumes, bread, cereals, rice and pasta.

Strangely, some people are more sensitive to low FODMAP ingredients than others (examples can include cornflour, lactose, wheat, starches, resistant starches - such as those found in reheated potato-, chillies, capsicum in bell peppers and many more). The individual nature of food tolerances is such that even if the food itself is low FODMAP some will experience discomfort. Unfortunately, the only way to identify these triggers is to test them and listen to the response your body gives, preferably under the assistance of a registered dietitian or nutritionist.

A low FODMAP jam is a jam which is made with a suitably low FODMAP fruit, such as raspberries or strawberries, and is made with sucrose or glucose syrup. High FODMAP jams have got added fructose, high fructose corn syrup, glucose-fructose syrup, honey, agave syrup, sorbitol, mannitol, xylitol, maltitol, erythritol and isomalt.

FODMAP stacking can occur when too many low FODMAP foods are included within one meal and inadvertently stack up to create a high FODMAP meal. Although some low FODMAP foods only have trace amounts of FODMAPs and can be pretty much eaten freely according to appetite, others are only low FODMAP in particular portion sizes. These portion-sized low FODMAP foods should be incorporated within our diets to ensure long-term health, but if you have too many of them in one meal you can stack up too many FODMAPs and give yourself digestive discomfort. However, all of the recipes in this book are low FODMAP as they are.

In summation, I would say that the most important thing to remember about the low FODMAP diet is that it is a low **FODMAP** diet, not a no **FODMAP** diet. As I always say, it's about making low FODMAP food good!

Bircher Muesli (Serves 1)

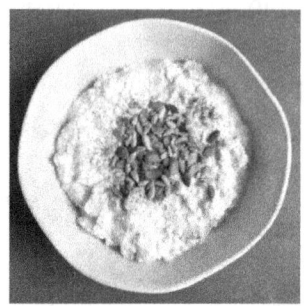

Ingredients:

40g gluten-free oats

1 small banana (chopped)

20g of Pink Lady or Granny Smith apple (diced or grated)

The zest of 1 navel orange (and some of the juice, if you like)

1/4 tsp ground cinnamon (add more to taste)

100g lactose-free natural yoghurt (or a non-dairy version)

100ml water

1 tsp pumpkin seeds

1 tsp sesame seeds

Method:
Simply prepare your ingredients as directed and mix together in a bowl. (I like to scatter my pumpkin and sesame seeds on top with a bit more cinnamon.)
Leave it overnight and then eat in the morning.
Bircher muesli is a lighter breakfast than overnight oats because it's made with 50% natural yoghurt (or a non-dairy option) and 50% water. It's also lighter because it contains grated apples. I know that apples have had a bad rap on the FODMAP street for a long time because initially Monash listed them as high

FODMAP, but they've been retested and now 20g portions of Pink Lady and Granny Smith apples are re-categorised as low FODMAP.

It's worth attempting to reintroduce apples because their flavour really adds a fresh crunch to the muesli bowl. Some people like to grate their apple into Bircher muesli, but I like to keep mine diced because it adds a gorgeous crunch to the muesli. Apples are also a brilliant source of fibre which helps to satisfy our good gut bacteria.

This Bircher muesli makes an excellent on-the-go breakfast and it's fresh, light and very nourishing. Go on, do a 'Snow White' and try the apple...

Orange And Ginger Compote

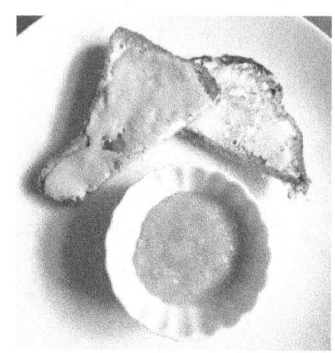

Ingredients:

370g oranges (peeled, deseeded and chopped)

20g fresh root ginger

8 tbsps. sugar

Method:
Put the chopped oranges and ginger in a NutriBullet, blender or food processor and blend until smooth before pouring it into a large saucepan and bringing to a simmer.
Add the sugar and stir until the sugar has dissolved.
Taste and add more sugar to suit your own tastes.
Once it's sweetened to your liking leave it to cool and then pour it into a clean jar or bowl and store it in the fridge.
I love fruit compotes because they're really versatile and are very handy to keep in the fridge to use on top of toast or porridge.
This orange and ginger compote has a delicious zingy freshness to it thanks to the use of sweet fresh oranges and it also packs a little heat in the form of fresh root ginger.
I like to blend it to a smooth jam-like consistency after I've made it, but you're welcome to keep it chunky if you prefer.

It's just a great low FODMAP fruit topping that'll keep for around a week in the fridge.
(You could also freeze it in small portions to defrost as required.)

Carrot And Orange Breakfast Bars (Makes 12)

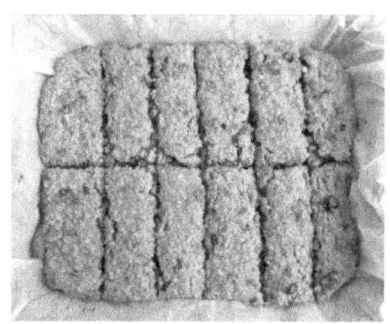

I created these breakfast bars one day when I wasn't in the mood for cereal or toast one morning, but I wanted something substantial and healthy to eat on the run for breakfasts during the week. The bars work really well as a quick breakfast because they are similar to baked oatmeal and when they're accompanied by a piece of fruit or a yoghurt they act as a very hearty meal with which to start your day. They're based on grated carrots, which ensure that the bars stay moist after they've been baked and they're infused with orange zest which provides a wonderful background citrus flavour. Actually, they're so tasty that I'll happily eat these bars at any time of the day! One bar is a low FODMAP portion.

Ingredients:

200g gluten-free rolled oats

170g grated carrots

1 mashed firm banana (around 110g)

The zest and juice of 1 orange

100g coconut oil

40g maple syrup

50g brown sugar

50g dried cranberries

1 tsp ground cinnamon

1 tsp vanilla extract

Method:
Preheat your oven to 180C/160C Fan/350F/Gas mark 4 and line a 25cm by 36cm (10" by 14") baking tin with greaseproof paper.
Put the coconut oil, maple syrup, brown sugar, vanilla extract and the zest and juice of the orange in a saucepan and gently heat it and stir it until the sugar has dissolved.
Put all of the other ingredients in a large mixing bowl and then pour the sugar mixture on top and stir it in well. Put the mixture into the greaseproofed baking tin and bake it for around 40-50 mins until it is golden brown.
Cut the lines you need to make it into bars while it is still warm, but leave it to cool completely in the tin before you remove the bars otherwise they can fall apart.

Baked Ham And Eggs (Serves 1-2)

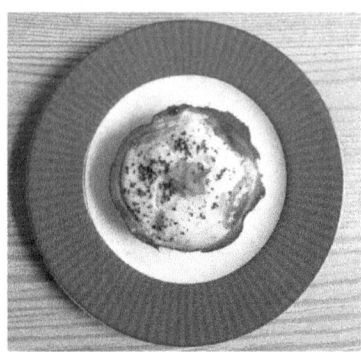

I love having baked ham and eggs for breakfast on weekends because they're very quick and easy to make, but are filling and indulgent at the same time.

They're formed by lining muffin tray holes with thick slices of cooked ham or bacon and then adding chopped peppers and tomatoes and cracking eggs on top and baking them.

As a result, the eggs are cooked within the ham 'liner' and become a self-enclosed breakfast.

They're tasty enough to eat just as they are, but you could also stretch them out to serve more people by serving them on top of slices of hot buttered toast.

Ingredients:

2 thick slices of cooked ham (or bacon)

2 eggs

¼ of a red bell pepper (chopped)

2 cherry tomatoes (cut into quarters)

Freshly ground black pepper

Fresh chopped chilli (optional)

Method:

Preheat your oven to 200C/180C Fan/400F/Gas mark 6.

Put the slices of ham into the tin you're using and press them down to form a bowl. Put the chopped bell pepper into the ham bowls and lie the tomato wedges in them.

Crack the eggs into the ham bowls and top with black pepper and chilli, if using.

Bake in the oven until the eggs are to your liking and then serve with or without hot buttered toast.

Low Fodmap Omelette (Serves 1)

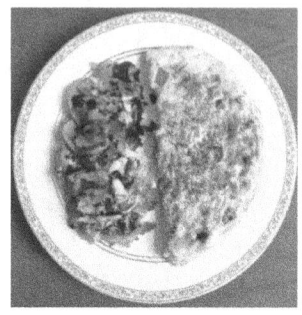

Ingredients:

2 eggs

30g lactose-free cheddar cheese (or non-dairy)

1 common tomato (finely diced)

10g chopped oyster mushroom

6 black olives (sliced)

1 tsp chopped chives

Freshly ground pepper

1 tbsp butter

I wanted to share this omelette recipe because sometimes I get sick of eating the same breakfasts over and over again. Toast. Porridge. Puffed rice. Granola. They just get tedious. That's what makes an omelette a great choice for mornings when you've got a bit more time on your hands and you can afford to spend some of it on making yourself a delicious breakfast for a change.

Omelettes are very simple meals which are based around a couple of whipped eggs, but you can make a myriad of omelette styles by adding a variety of ingredients to the egg base. I make mine with cheese, tomato, black olives and oyster mushrooms, but you could also add chopped cooked meat, such as ham, chicken or even salmon. You can also add chopped red or green bell peppers, jalapeños or chopped fresh chillies to the mix too.

I like to serve my omelettes with a side salad because they're quite filling, but if you were really hungry you could supplement them with a couple of slices of hot buttered toast. It's also worth bearing in mind that omelettes are a brilliant quick evening meal for when you need something speedy for dinner and they also pair wonderfully with a side serving of hot salted chips.

Method:

Crack your eggs into a bowl and whisk them with a fork until they are light and fluffy.

Add all of your ingredients (except the butter) and whisk together.

Put a non-stick frying pan over a low to medium heat and put the tablespoon of butter in it. Once the butter has melted pour the omelette mixture into the frying pan.

Let it gently cook until it is almost completely done, but it still has a bit of wobble in the middle and then gently fold one half of the omelette over the other to form a half moon shape. Cook for a minute or two more before serving.

Butternut Squash And Mixed Spice Muffins (Makes 12)

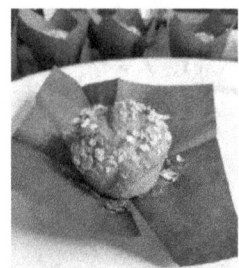

Ingredients:

350g peeled and diced butternut squash (prepared weight)

120g sugar

4 eggs

200g gluten-free self-raising flour

1 tsp baking powder

1 tsp xanthan gum

1 tsp mixed spice

150ml vegetable oil

The zest of 1 orange

30g rolled porridge oats

Some mornings are made for leisurely breakfasts, such as these Butternut Squash and Mixed Spice Muffins. Mornings of this nature include weekends and holidays. Days when you have a bit more time to dedicate to making something for your breakfast which is utterly delicious and just a little bit decadent. These muffins are one such breakfast option which are a bit more time-consuming to create, but are massively rewarding in the taste department.

If I know the night before that I'm going to make these muffins for breakfast the following morning I tend to steam the butternut squash in advance so that it's cool by morning in order to cut out a step, but if you take the notion on the morning in question to make them it's not that big a deal to cook the squash then. These muffins are only slightly sweet, allowing you to have the option of either serving them as they are or with a dollop of butter on top. One muffin is a low FODMAP serving.

Method:

Preheat your oven to 200C/180C Fan/400F/Gas Mark 6 and put 12 cases in a muffin tray.

Peel the butternut squash and cut it into small chunks of around 2cm square. Cook them on a plate in a microwave until soft and leave to cool. (If you don't have a microwave you can just roast the cubes until they are soft.)

Put all of your ingredients (except for the oats) into a large mixing bowl and mix together well. (It's fine to leave chunks of whole squash.)

Divide the mixture between the 12 muffin cases and then scatter the oats on top.

Bake in the oven for 25-30 mins or until a skewer pushed into the middle of one comes out clean.

Remove from the oven and serve. Butter is optional, but recommended, as always!

Kedgeree (Serves 2)

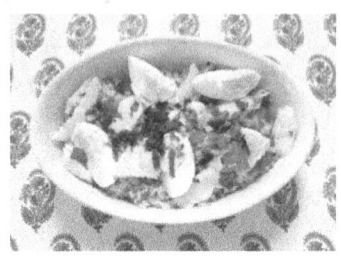

Ingredients:

300g smoked haddock

4 eggs

150g rice

1 tbsp coconut oil

1 tsp ground turmeric

1 tbsp fresh ginger (minced)

1-2 tbsps of mild curry powder

2 common tomatoes (chopped)

1/4 of a red chilli (finely chopped, but optional)

Lactose-free natural yoghurt (or dairy-free version) & fresh coriander leaves

Kedgeree is an Indian breakfast which consists of spiced rice, smoked haddock and hard-boiled eggs. It might sound like an odd choice for breakfast because, let's be honest, not many of us would reach for rice and smoked haddock first thing in the morning, but trust me when I say that this is well worth making at least once.

Although smoked haddock is traditionally used in kedgeree, you could replace it with tuna or salmon, should you prefer and if you want to save time you could cook the eggs the day before and use microwaveable ready-cooked rice pouches.

Kedgeree might not be a conventional breakfast, but it's a very tasty one. Its beauty lies in its tender yellow grains of turmeric-infused long grain rice, its generous chunks of tender flaked smoked haddock and quartered, hard-boiled creamy eggs, all of which is encased in the fresh flavours of minced ginger and traditional curry spices. It's an unexpected, but firm breakfast favourite of mine now!

Method:

In a bowl, mix the chopped coriander leaves into the natural yoghurt and leave to one side.

Put the eggs in a saucepan of boiling water and boil the eggs for around 8 minutes. Drain the eggs and top the saucepan up with cold water. Once the eggs are cool enough to handle peel them, cut the eggs into quarters and leave to one side.

Cook the haddock in a frying pan under water until firm. Leave to cool and then cut into chunks.

Boil the rice with the turmeric until the rice is tender and then drain.

Melt the coconut oil in a frying pan and once it's melted add the minced ginger, curry powder and sliced tomatoes. Fry until the tomatoes are soft.

Add the rice and haddock to the pan and heat through. Add the chilli (if using) and then add the quartered eggs. Serve with dollops of the yoghurt and fresh coriander leaves.

Shakshuka (Serves 2-4)

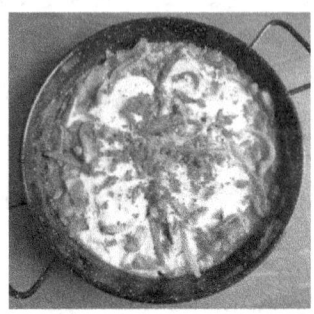

When I put a call out to my friends a while ago for recipes that they'd like to see featured on my blog one of my friends asked me to make shakshuka. (Sorry it's taken so long, Chiara!) Shakshuka is a breakfast dish which originates from the Mediterranean and Middle East and is composed of eggs which are baked on a bed of sliced bell peppers that are cooked in a rich and spicy tomato sauce.

At first I didn't really fancy the idea of eggs baked in spicy peppers for breakfast because it seemed a bit adventurous for first thing in the morning, but I gave it a go for a late breakfast one morning and was blown away with how tasty it actually is. I added smoked bacon to my shakshuka because bacon's delicious and enhances the flavour of everything it meets, but feel free to leave it out if you prefer.

Shakshuka is filled with flavour. The sweet sliced bell peppers are gently cooked along with smoked bacon pieces in the spiced chopped tomatoes to form a flavoursome base upon which the eggs are baked. You can have this for breakfast, brunch or even dinner and you won't be disappointed.

Ingredients:

1 tsp coconut oil

4 rashers of smoked bacon (chopped)

2 red or green bell peppers (cored and sliced)

4 eggs

2 tbsps. chopped chives

1 tsp sweet paprika

1/2 tsp ground cumin

180g tinned chopped tomatoes

Fresh coriander leaves and fresh chopped chilli

Method:
Preheat your oven to 200C/180C Fan/400F/Gas mark 6.
Put a large frying pan over a medium heat and melt the coconut oil in it before adding the bacon and peppers.
Once the bacon is cooked add the spices and chopped tomatoes and then put the mixture in an ovenproof casserole dish.
Make 4 small wells in the shakshuka and crack your eggs into them.
Bake the shakshuka in the oven until the eggs are cooked to your liking before serving it with fresh coriander and sliced fresh chilli.

Quinoa Porridge (Serves 1)

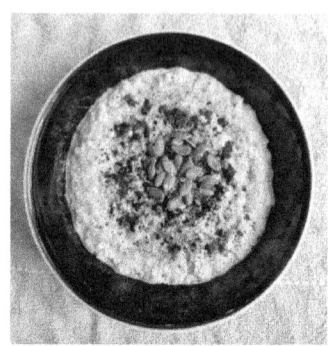

Quinoa porridge is a very tasty alternative to oats because quinoa has a unique 'nutty' texture.

It's also packed with protein which keeps your appetite at bay for a long time. I first made this porridge without soaking the quinoa overnight, but it takes way less time to make if you soak it because it's much quicker to cook.

And, if you like, you can add a teaspoon of cocoa powder to your porridge which will give it a gorgeous chocolatey flavour.

I'd really encourage any porridge aficionado to try quinoa porridge at least once because it's healthy, hearty and very, very tasty.

Ingredients:

50g quinoa

200g lactose-free milk (or non-dairy)

1 tbsp chia seeds

Sugar (to taste)

Method:

Put the quinoa and chia seeds in a saucepan and soak them in the milk overnight.

In the morning put the saucepan over a medium heat and simmer it until the quinoa is soft.

Add a bit of boiling water if you feel it is getting too thick.

Once you're happy with the softness of the quinoa add sugar to taste and once it's dissolved serve.

Breakfast Burgers (Makes 2)

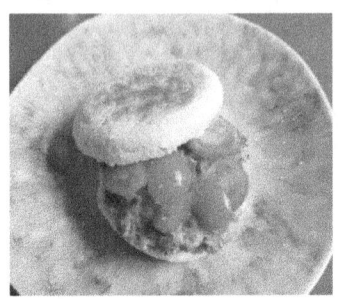

Ingredients:

200g pork mince

1/2 tsp dried sage

1/2 tsp dried thyme

1/4 tsp ground black pepper

1/4 tsp salt

1/4 tsp dried rosemary

1 tsp dried parsley

1 tbsp vegetable oil

2 gluten-free English muffins

2 slices of lactose-free cheese

(or non-dairy)

As much as I enjoy sausages for breakfast, sometimes it's nice to have something a bit different. That's where these breakfast burgers come in.

A well-known fast-food company sells tasty breakfast muffins and I thought it'd be nice to make a similar herb-infused breakfast burger to enjoy within a gluten-free English muffin.

After a bit of experimentation with the herb levels I ended up with a burger which had just the right ratio of seasoning to pork mince.

I like to serve mine with slices of fresh tomato, but you could top it with a fried egg or poached egg, if you like. A rasher or two of bacon never goes amiss either.

Method:

Mix all of the seasonings into the pork mince until it is well combined and then form the mince into two thin burger patties.

Heat the oil in a frying pan and fry the breakfast burgers until they are fully cooked through.

While they are cooking toast the muffins and if you're having eggs with them make them too.

Serve the breakfast burgers inside the buttered muffin.

Breakfast Chimichangas (Serves 1)

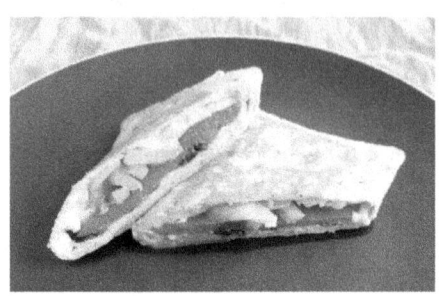

I'm a big fan of chimichangas because I love the crispy toasted flavour of the lightly fried tortilla which encases a delicious filling. They might not seem like an obvious choice for breakfast, but trust me when I say that they make for a very tasty breakfast or brunch.

I love jars of roasted red bell peppers in brine because not only are they low FODMAP, they're very handy to add to sandwiches, pizzas and chimichangas.

I like to fill my chimichangas with cheese, olives, jalapeños and a bit of both jarred roasted red peppers and chopped fresh yellow bell pepper too, so that the soft texture of the roasted pepper contrasts with the crunchy crisp fresh pepper.

Ingredients:

1 gluten-free wrap or corn tortilla

1 tsp oil

30g grated cheddar cheese (or a non-dairy version)

¼ of a fresh yellow bell pepper (chopped)

Half a jarred roasted red pepper (well-drained)

2 black olives (sliced)

Jalapeños (optional)

Freshly ground black pepper

Method:

Heat the oil in a frying pan over a medium heat. Lay the tortilla flat and place the cheese in the centre of it before adding the rest of your filling.

Fold the sides into the middle so they touch and then fold the top and bottom into the middle so that a tight parcel is formed.

Place the tortilla fold-side down in the frying pan and fry until the base is golden brown and crispy. Turn it over and toast the other side too. Once it's toasted remove it from the frying pan and serve.

Soups

Soups

P.30 - Tomato and Carrot

P.31 - Curried Coconut and Parsnip

P.32 - Winter Vegetable Broth

P.33 - Carrot and Coconut

P.34 - Minestrone

P.35 - Cream of Mushroom

P.36 - Chicken Soup

P.37 - Fish Chowder

P.38 - Potato and Chive Soup

P.39 - Butternut Squash and Ginger

Tomato And Carrot Soup (Serves 2)

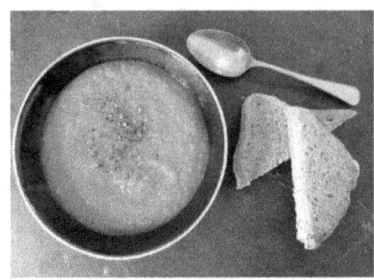

One day I was looking in the fridge and I noticed that the back of my fridge was frozen. I turned the thermostat down and didn't give it more thought until the following week when I started noticing that the fridge had begun to freeze everything that was sitting near the back of it. Needless to say, I needed a new fridge. The problem was I hadn't long done a decent-sized food shop, so it was filled with fresh vegetables that I certainly wasn't going to throw out! Instead, I popped the vegetables in my freezer and within a few days this soup recipe was born.

I paired the tomatoes with a couple of carrots (which were also casualties of the fridge-freezing incident) and a couple of low FODMAP stock cubes and a very delicious and warming soup was created. The natural sweetness of the carrots and the zingy, slightly tart, tang of the fresh tomatoes complement each other really well and they are enhanced by the inclusion of fresh thyme leaves. It's now become one of my favourite homemade soups!

Ingredients:

8 common tomatoes (diced)

2 large carrots (peeled and thinly sliced)

2 low FODMAP vegetable stock cubes

300-500ml boiling water (depending on how thick you want your soup)

Method:

Place your prepared vegetables, stock cubes and boiling water in a large saucepan and bring it to the boil. Simmer your soup for 10-15 mins until the carrots are soft.

If you'd like a smooth soup use a food processor, **HAND-HELD BLENDER** or NutriBullet to blend your soup until smooth, but exercise caution with the hot soup. Serve.

Curried Coconut And Parsnip (Serves 4-6)

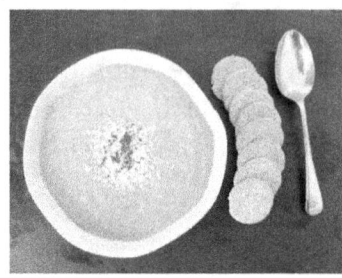

Parsnips are an incredibly flavoursome FODMAP-free vegetable and they naturally have quite a creamy, sweet taste, so I thought it would be nice to enhance these qualities further by blending parsnips with a base of creamy coconut milk to create a silky, decadent soup.

The inclusion of garam masala spice cuts through the sweetness of the soup and adds a lovely spiciness which prevents it from being too cloying.

I like this soup blended smooth, so that all of the flavours meld together, but you can leave the parsnips chunky, if you prefer, to have a heartier soup. The choice is entirely yours.

Ingredients:

700g parsnips (peeled and chopped)

320g tinned coconut milk

2 tsps. garam masala

1 pint of vegetable stock

Salt and pepper

Method:

Put all of the ingredients into a large saucepan and bring to the boil.

Simmer until the parsnips are soft.

Blend until smooth and then season to taste and serve.

Winter Vegetable Broth (Serves 4)

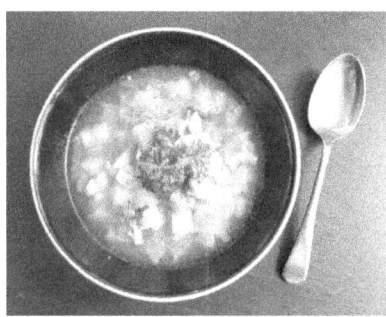

At the end of summer when the weather turns and the jewel-coloured leaves start their gentle cascade to the ground I start getting excited because I know that cosy evenings are waiting just around the corner.

Being a winter baby, my world is rocked not by heat, sunshine and tans, but lit candles, fleece throws, quality autumn and winter TV shows, Jack Frost leaving his unique graffiti all over everything he touches overnight, and hot candlelit baths before early nights tucked up in bed with a really good book.

And let's not forget the food-based delights that cold weather brings, such as hearty stews, warming sweet puddings and simple, yet delicious, bowls of hot soup, such as this winter vegetable broth. Sunshine worshippers are welcome to it, in my opinion.

Ingredients:

1000ml vegetable stock

160g diced carrot

100g diced parsnip

150g diced potato

40g sliced common cabbage

50g broccoli heads (cut small)

10g green spring onion tips

¼ tsp dried thyme

¼ tsp dried rosemary

Method:
Prepare the vegetables as directed and put all of them along with the thyme in a saucepan with the stock.
Bring to the boil and cook until the vegetables are tender.
Season to taste and serve with crusty bread.

Carrot And Coconut Soup (Serves 2)

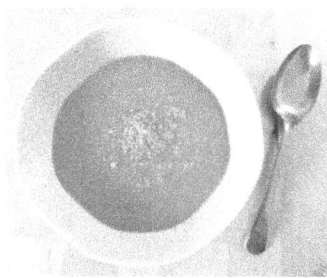

Carrot and coconut soup is a real winner in my eyes because the carrots provide a wonderful sweetness and smooth texture to the soup while the coconut milk makes it silky and creamy on the tongue.

The question of whether to blend or not to blend is up to you to answer, but I like to add a little bit of background spice in the form of ground cumin and turmeric to my soup, but you can just keep it plain, if you'd prefer.

Whether you add the spice or not it's light, fresh and flavoursome. Your sandwiches are crying out to be dunked in this soup!

Ingredients:

320g carrots (peeled and grated)

160g tinned coconut milk

500ml vegetable stock

¼ tsp ground cumin

¼ tsp ground turmeric

Salt and pepper to taste

Method:

Put all of your ingredients in a large saucepan and bring it to the boil.

Simmer until the carrots are soft and blend if you like. Season to taste and serve.

Minestrone (Serves 4)

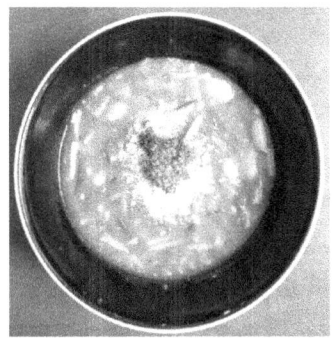

Minestrone soup is a classic Italian soup made from a fresh tomato base which surrounds a variety of vegetable, beans and pasta shapes (all of which differ depending on who you're talking to). Quite frankly, it's a meal in itself! Its status is iconic because it's got something in it for everyone and tends to hold universal appeal. This minestrone recipe may be simple, but it's fresh, filling and full of flavour. It's the perfect lunch or evening meal and you could even make this in your slow cooker throughout the day, if you like.

Ingredients:

1 large carrot (peeled and diced)

360g tinned chopped tomatoes

60g gluten-free spaghetti (broken into 1 inch pieces)

400ml vegetable stock

80g green beans (cut into small pieces)

120g butter beans (drained and rinsed well)

1/2 tsp dried oregano

2 tbsps chopped chives

Fresh parsley or basil leaves

20g grated parmesan (or non-dairy version)

Method:

Keeping the parmesan and fresh herbs to one side, put all of your prepared ingredients in a large pot and bring to a gentle simmer, stirring occasionally to make sure nothing sticks to the bottom of the pot.

Once your pasta and vegetables are tender you can serve it scattered with the fresh herbs and parmesan.

Cream Of Mushroom Soup (Serves 2)

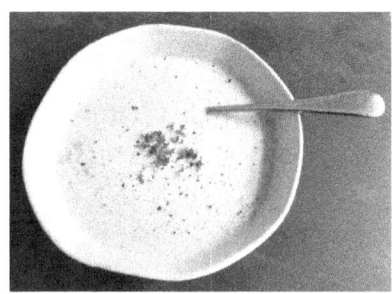

Mushrooms tend to be high FODMAP, but oyster mushrooms are delightfully low FODMAP in servings of less than 75g per person, so they're ideal for using in this recipe. I like to add fresh thyme leaves to my soup because it's quite a deep, 'woody'-flavoured herb which goes very well with the earthy flavour of the mushrooms, but if you're not a fan of thyme feel free to leave it out. (If you use dried thyme leaves only add 1/2 a teaspoon because they're much stronger than fresh leaves.)

This cream of mushroom soup is quite thin as opposed to many of the thick soups I tend to make, but it's no less for it because it's extremely flavoursome and rich. I also quite like the fact that it's so thin because you can drink it out of a cup without seeming uncouth! If you're a mushroom lover who's looking for a simple, but very tasty soup to make in next to no time at all then this is one for you.

Ingredients:

140g oyster mushrooms (thinly sliced)

2 FODMAP-friendly vegetable stock cubes

600ml boiling water

2 tsps fresh thyme leaves (optional)

100ml lactose-free double cream (or non-dairy version)

Salt and pepper to taste

Method:

Dissolve the stock into the boiling water.

Put a saucepan over a medium heat and add the mushrooms, thyme and stock.

Bring to the boil and simmer for 5-10 minutes until the mushrooms are soft.

Remove from the heat and add the double cream and stir.

Blend the soup until smooth and then serve.

Chicken Soup (Serves 4)

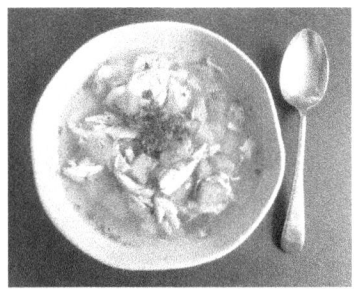

There are few things in this world which are as restorative and comforting as chicken soup and this is a particularly tasty one thanks to the use of fresh herbs. I like to make mine with fresh chicken stock, partly because of the sheer punch of flavour it adds and partly because it tends to be free from pesky added FODMAPs, such as onion and garlic. I also like to use shredded cooked chicken that's left over from a roast because I think the flavour is far superior to that which comes from plain old chicken breasts, but it's totally up to you. Regardless, you'll create a potful of comforting, soothing and warming broth.

Ingredients:

350g cooked chicken (shredded)

2-3 carrots (peeled and diced)

1 litre of chicken stock

2 tbsps of fresh parsley (chopped)

1 tsp fresh thyme leaves

1 tbsp butter (or non-dairy)

Salt and pepper

Method:
Melt the butter in a large saucepan and add the diced carrots and fry them until they are soft.

Add the chicken stock, herbs and shredded cooked chicken. Cook until the soup is hot and then season to taste and serve.

Fish Chowder (Serves 2-4)

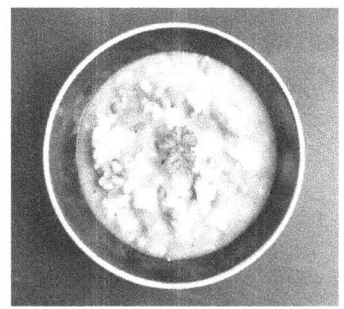

Ingredients:

2 tbsps. butter (or non-dairy)

1 tbsp. gluten-free plain flour

400ml fish or vegetable stock

2 tbsps. chopped fresh chives

130g cubed potato

60g cubed carrot

2 common tomatoes (diced)

120g cod, haddock or salmon (cut into chunks)

100g cooked prawns

30g garden peas

1 tbsp. fresh chopped parsley

Salt and pepper to taste

Although many people might think that you'd need to be a real fan of fish and seafood to enjoy this soup they'd be wrong because it's not actually overly 'fishy' tasting. It is however, a very delicious and somewhat decadent soup which makes for quite a treat at the dinner table.

You can add clams or mussels to this soup, if you like, and you can also use smoked fish, if preferred. It might seem like an odd addition, but an optional ingredient which adds a lot of flavour to this soup is a couple of rashers of bacon because it infuses the soup with a real background richness. (Smoked bacon is particularly good).

And, as with all soups, you can add more stock if you prefer a thinner consistency.

Method:

Put the butter in a large saucepan over a medium heat and once it's melted add the tablespoon of flour and cook it for a couple of minutes, stirring all the while.

Slowly add the stock, a little at a time, until a smooth sauce is formed.

Add the chives, potato, carrot and tomatoes and cook until the potato is soft.

Add the fish, peas and prawns and cook until the fish is cooked through and flaky.

Serve scattered with the freshly chopped parsley.

Potato And Chive Soup (Serves 4)

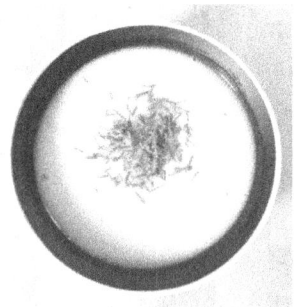

I'm going to be honest, when I initially set out to make a standard potato soup I didn't really think it was going to be particularly mind-blowing, but, good grief, was I proved wrong when I tasted it! The beauty of this soup lies in the use of new potatoes as opposed to old potatoes because the new potatoes are so inherently buttery that they elevate the creaminess of the soup to the extent that you'd be forgiven for thinking that there was half a pound of butter added to it! If I could implore you to make one soup from this chapter it'd definitely be this one, my friends!

Ingredients:

500g new potatoes

800ml chicken stock (or vegetable stock, if preferred)

200ml lactose-free cream or non-dairy milk

10g fresh chopped chives

Salt and pepper to taste

Method:
Remove any spots on the potato skins, so they are clean and then cut them into small chunks and put them in a large pan.

Add the chicken stock and most of the chives (reserving a little bit of chopped chives for decoration, if you like) and bring to the boil.

Cook until the potatoes are soft and then add the cream or milk and blend well until smooth.

Taste for seasoning and serve with the chopped chives on top.

Butternut Squash And Ginger (Serves 4)

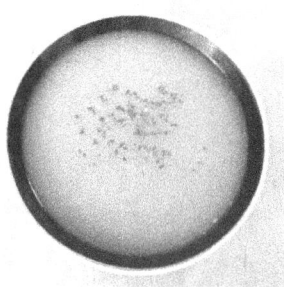

As much as I tend to prefer chunky soups I also sometimes like a thinner broth because I've learned that just because a soup has a more watery texture it doesn't necessarily have to mean that the flavour is watered down. This soup is a perfect case in point because although it's thin enough to drink it from a mug (and please do, I won't judge you) it's incredibly flavoursome. The earthy sweetness of the butternut squash melds perfectly with the root ginger to produce a soup that's filling and has just the right amount of background heat. It's perfect for sandwich dunking.

Ingredients:

180g butternut squash (prepared weight)

200g potato (prepared weight)

15g minced fresh ginger

500ml low FODMAP vegetable stock

Salt and pepper (to taste)

Method:
Peel and de-seed the butternut squash and cut it into small chunks.
Peel the potatoes and cut them into small chunks.

Place the vegetables, ginger and stock in a large pan and bring to the boil. Once the vegetables are soft taste and season the soup with salt and pepper.

Blend the soup until smooth and feel free to add more water to loosen the texture if you like.

Serve.

Light meals, lunches and snacks

Light Meals, Lunches and Snacks

P.42 - Roasted New Potato Salad

P.43 - Taquitos

P.44 - Caprese Bruschetta

P.45 - Halloumi Fries

P.46 - Chicken Burritos

P.47 - Gluten-Free Pizzas

P.48 - Dirty Fries

P.49 - Popcorn Chicken

P.50 - Cornish Pasties

P.51 - Spiced Sweet Potato and Feta Wraps

P.52 - Vegetable Samosas

P.53 - Roasted Red Pepper and Tomato Salad

Roasted New Potato Salad (Serves 1)

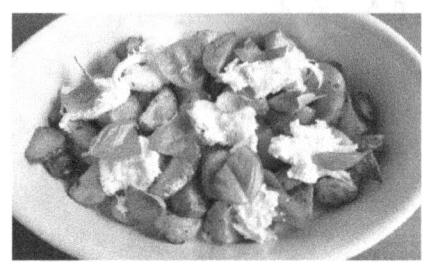

Salads aren't something that I reach for very often and my waistline often laments it, but I'm a big fan of this roasted new potato salad because it's so substantial. The fact that it contains chunks of torn creamy mozzarella is undoubtedly a major factor too.

I made this salad for one person because it's easy enough to increase the total quantities in order to accommodate extra diners, should you need to. Since developing this recipe my family has enjoyed it both hot and cold for lunches and dinners and it never fails to be a hit. Give it a whirl and see what you think!

Ingredients:

Enough new potatoes for one person

1 tbsp vegetable oil

1/2 tsp dried oregano

40g mozzarella or feta cheese (or a non-dairy version)

3 cherry tomatoes (cut into wedges)

1 or 2 gherkins (sliced)

1-2 tsps of red wine vinegar

Fresh basil leaves

Salt and pepper

Method:

Preheat your oven to 200C/180C Fan/400F/Gas mark 6.

Cut the potatoes into bite-sized pieces and put them into a baking tin and add the oregano and salt and pepper. Coat them in the vegetable oil and roast them until they are tender in the middle.

Leave them to cool and then mix all of the salad components together and serve.

Taquitos (Serves 4)

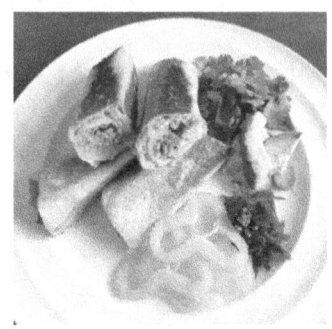

Ingredients:

400g beef mince

6 rashers of smoked back bacon (chopped)

100g green bell pepper (diced)

1 tsp ground cumin

1 tbsp smoked paprika

3 tbsps vegetable oil

150g grated cheddar cheese (or non-dairy version)

8 corn tortillas (or gluten-free tortillas)

If you don't know what taquitos are, they're basically a tortilla wrap that's filled with tasty ingredients, wrapped up like a cigar and then fried in a little oil to create a crispy tube that encases its filling.

I make mine with minced beef, but you can easily make them vegetarian or vegan by using grated cheddar cheese (or a non-dairy version) and a selection of low FODMAP vegetables instead.

I tend to make these for lunch, but they're substantial enough to serve them for dinner with either salad on the side or rice.

Method:

Put 1 tbsp of oil in a large saucepan and fry the beef and bacon with the spices and green pepper until cooked.

Remove from the heat and get a frying pan ready.

Lay your tortilla out and put some cheese on it followed by some of the beef mix and roll into a cigar shape. Put some vegetable oil in the frying pan over a medium heat and once it's hot put your taquitos in folded edge down.

Fry the taquitos on their folded edge until they have browned underneath and then gently turn the taquitos over to brown them and crisp them up all over.

Keep your cooked taquitos in a warm oven until you have cooked all of the taquitos and then serve with salad and freshly chopped coriander.

Caprese Bruschetta (Serves 2)

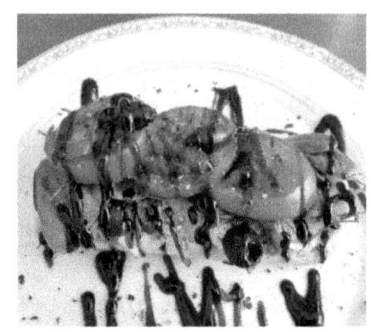

Ingredients:

2 gluten-free panini rolls (halved horizontally)

120g mozzarella (sliced) (or a non-dairy version)

2 common tomatoes (thinly sliced)

10 English spinach leaves

Fresh basil leaves (to suit your own taste)

2 tbsps of balsamic glaze or vinegar (use less, if preferred)

1 tbsp extra virgin olive oil

2 tbsps fresh chives (finely chopped)

10 pitted black olives (halved)

Black pepper

Freshly chopped red chilli (optional)

Bruschetta is a traditional Italian antipasto (starter) dish which can be traced back to ancient Rome. It's normally made from toasted bread which is rubbed with garlic and salt and is then drizzled with olive oil before being topped with vegetables, meat and cheese.

This recipe for caprese bruschetta celebrates every single aspect of the individual components which make it up: the tangy, sweet tomatoes; the soft, aromatic freshly torn basil leaves; the tart, but sweet, vinegar component of the balsamic glaze; and the soft yeasty toasted ciabatta roll it all sits on top of.

It's fresh, light and incredibly tasty.

Method:

Prepare your ingredients as directed.

Toast your buns lightly and once they're done layer the mozzarella and salad ingredients on top in whatever order you like.

Drizzle with the balsamic glaze or balsamic vinegar and give it a good scattering of freshly ground black pepper before serving.

Halloumi Fries (Serves 2)

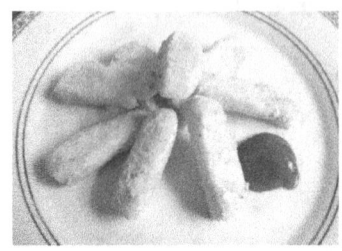

Ingredients:

80g of halloumi cheese

3 tbsps of gluten-free plain flour

1/4 tsp ground black pepper

1/2 tsp ground sweet paprika

Halloumi fries are a great idea because how do you improve on the tasty snack that is fries? Make them out of cheese, of course! Joking aside, halloumi fries are seriously tasty and are an excellent side dish to serve alongside meals.

Halloumi is a firm cheese which originates from Cyprus and has a very high melting point. As a result, the beauty of halloumi is that it doesn't melt when you cook it and it holds its shape, making it ideal for crafting things like fries out of it.

Halloumi is quite unique in that due to its firm texture it has a 'squeaky' aspect to it upon chewing. If you've never eaten halloumi before that probably sounds like quite an odd quality to the cheese, but trust me, it's delicious.

It's quite a salty cheese, so although I add ground black pepper to the coating I never add salt because it's simply not needed. If you'd like them to have a bit of a spice kick you can easily add 1/4 tsp of ground chilli powder to the flour coating. Another option is to use smoked paprika instead of sweet paprika because it will give the fries a smoky flavour.

These fries are really rewarding in taste. The firm, creamy halloumi is coated in delicately seasoned gluten-free flour and upon baking they're simply begging to have their crispy little selves dunked in good ketchup.

Method:

Preheat your oven to 200C/180C Fan/400F/Gas mark 6.

Measure out 80g of halloumi and cut the halloumi into fry-shaped sticks.

Mix the flour, black pepper and paprika together on a plate and then toss the halloumi sticks in it until they are fully coated.

Place them on a baking tray and bake them in the oven until they are golden brown. Serve.

Chicken Burritos (Serves 4)

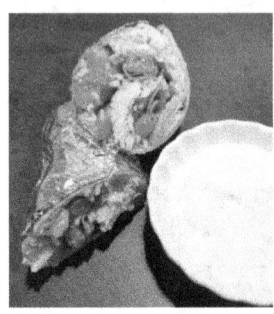

Ingredients for the chicken:

3 chicken breasts (thinly sliced)

1 red bell pepper (thinly sliced)

2 tsps smoked paprika

2 tsps ground cumin

1/4 tsp dried ground chilli (optional)

1 tbsp vegetable oil

The juice of 1 lime

Accompaniments:

A pouch of ready-cooked Tilda coconut rice (or ready-cooked plain rice)

4 gluten-free tortilla wraps

Fresh coriander (chopped)

2 sliced common tomatoes

Shredded iceberg lettuce

100g grated mozzarella or cheddar (or non-dairy version)

The best burrito I ever ate was in a burrito restaurant in Edinburgh. My step-daughter had insisted we go there for lunch and although I didn't expect the food to be astronomical I agreed to her suggestion. I had a huge, soft duvet-like tortilla that was stuffed to the gunnels with Mexican rice, re-fried beans, salsa, guacamole, and tender strips of chicken. Aww, man! It was heaven wrapped in tinfoil.

I've no doubt that the chicken burrito I just described was in no way low FODMAP, so I set about creating the right combination of ingredients which would ensure that I could recreate the heavenly burrito in question. I'm glad to report that my quest was successful, producing the recipe I'm happy to share below.

My chicken burrito recipe incorporates a soft gluten-free tortilla that surrounds tender grains of rice, piquant grated cheddar cheese, fresh salad leaves and tender pieces of chicken breast. It's a great treat at lunchtime, but it can also serve as a quick and light evening meal too.

Method:

Put a large saucepan over a medium heat and add the oil before adding the sliced chicken, spices and lime juice.

Fry the chicken for 5 mins before adding the sliced red pepper and continuing to cook it for another 10 mins or until the chicken is fully cooked.

To make your burrito place your tortilla on a flat surface and put your chosen ingredients in a line down the centre.

Fold the sides in towards the middle until they overlap the edge of the burrito filling, then take the side closest to you and fold it over the filling before wrapping it completely. Serve.

Gluten-Free Pizzas (Serves 1)

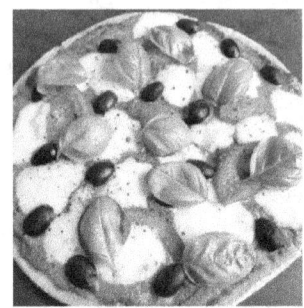

I absolutely adore pizzas because they're a brilliant base upon which to serve a wide range of delicious toppings, but although toppings are important, one of the things which makes a good pizza is its base. Now, the texture of this pizza base isn't the same as a standard gluten one because, quite frankly, the properties of gluten are pretty much impossible to replicate, but this is a great alternative because it holds its shape well, works as a perfect carrier surface for delicious pizza toppings, and it's very tasty too.

I base my dough around the traditional raising agent baking powder which has the same effect as yeast, but takes far less time to work. I also lightly cook the base prior to putting the toppings on. For a long time I thought pizza was permanently off the menu on the low FODMAP diet because I couldn't eat wheat, so this recipe was a revelation! I hope you think so too.

Ingredients:

200g self-raising gluten-free flour (plus a little more for dusting & rolling the dough)

160g lactose-free natural yoghurt

¼ tsp salt

½ tsp baking powder

¼ tsp xanthan gum

Method:

Preheat your oven to 200C/180C Fan/400F/Gas mark 6 and lay a flour-dusted sheet of greaseproof paper on top of your work surface.

Mix all of the ingredients together in a large bowl and then roll the dough out on top of the greaseproof until it is around ½ a centimetre thick.

Bake the pizza base in the oven for 15-20 mins until it is lightly browned and then add your pizza sauce and toppings and bake it again until your toppings are cooked. Serve.

Dirty Fries (Serves 2-4)

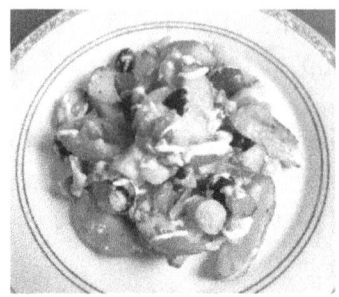

Ingredients:

Enough potatoes for however many people you're feeding (roughly 300-400g per person)

1-2 tbsps vegetable oil

1 sliced green bell pepper

70g sliced pickled gherkins

60g sliced black olives

80g lactose-free grated cheddar cheese (or a non-dairy version)

1 common tomato (cut into thin wedges)

4 low FODMAP sausages (thinly sliced)

Jalapenos or fresh chilli (optional)

Although I love eating Dirty Fries, I strongly object to their name because there's nothing particularly 'dirty' about them! They're referred to as 'dirty' because they're topped with traditionally 'naughty' foods, such as melted cheddar cheese, but the fact of the matter is, there's nothing wrong with incorporating sensible portions of cheese within a healthy diet.

There's also absolutely nothing wrong with eating fries as such, as long as they're not drenched in oil. In fact, potatoes are an excellent source of vitamins B6 and C, so they're a brilliant addition to our diets.

These Dirty Fries make an absolutely awesome evening meal and they're seriously popular with kids and teenagers. I think they're particularly good because every mouthful is a different flavour combination and they make a delicious vegetarian option for dinner if you leave out the sausage. However you choose to top your Dirty Fries you certainly won't feel dirty after eating them!

Method:

Preheat your oven to 200C/180C Fan/400F/Gas Mark 6.

Wash your potatoes (and peel them if preferred) before cutting them into equal wedges.

Place them on a large baking tray and coat them in the vegetable oil before sprinkling them with freshly ground pepper. (I tend not to add salt because the cheddar cheese adds salt anyway.)

Bake the fries in the oven until they are just tender (around 30-40 mins) and then top the fries with all of the other ingredients before scattering the cheddar cheese on top.

Cook the dirty fries in the oven until the sausage is cooked through and the cheese is melted and golden brown. Serve.

Popcorn Chicken (Serves 2-4)

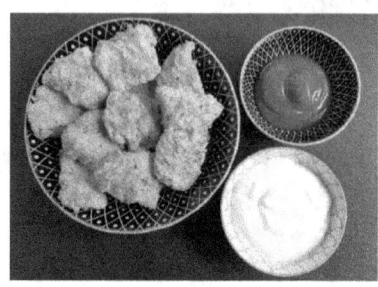

Popcorn chicken is a seriously tasty bite-sized snack which makes a refreshing change for lunch rather than the standard sandwich. They are, in essence, chicken nuggets, but they have a delicious seasoned coating which differentiates them from a standard nugget. You can use smoked paprika instead of sweet paprika if you'd like a smokier flavour and you can also add dried ground chilli powder if you'd like a spicy kick. They're particularly gorgeous dipped in my **LEMON MAYO** recipe which can be found in the **FISH CHAPTER**.

Ingredients:

2 chicken breasts (cut into bite-sized pieces)

4 tbsps gluten-free flour

1/2 a tsp of salt

1/4 tsp ground black pepper

1 tsp sweet paprika

1 tsp dried oregano

1 egg

1 tbsp lemon juice

Method:
Preheat your oven to 200C/180C Fan/400F/Gas Mark 6 and have a baking tray at hand.

Cut the chicken into bite-sized pieces.
Put the flour and seasonings into a low sided bowl and mix together.
Put the egg and lemon juice in another bowl and whisk it together.
Dip the chicken pieces in the egg and then into the flour before placing them on a baking tray. Once all of the chicken pieces have been coated bake them in the oven for 10-12 mins until the chicken pieces are no longer pink in the middle.
Serve with lemon mayo and ketchup.

Cornish Pasties (Makes 6)

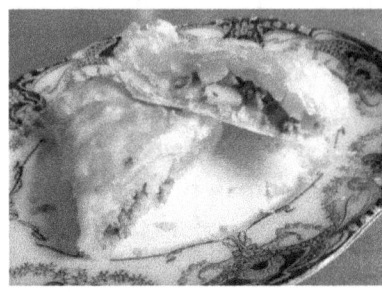

Cornish pasties are a great lunch option, particularly if you're looking for something substantial to take as a packed lunch. They're traditionally made with beef skirt, a lean and tender cut of beef, but it's expensive, so I tend to just use mince instead. They're also normally made with shortcrust pastry, but it's hard to find a gluten-free version, so I just make mine with gluten-free puff pastry instead and I think they're just as tasty. Feel free to make them with whichever you prefer though.

Ingredients:

500g gluten-free puff pastry

200g beef mince

100g turnip/swede (peeled and diced into 1cm chunks)

100g carrots (peeled and diced into 1cm chunks)

200g potatoes (peeled and diced into 1cm chunks)

1/2 tsp black pepper

1 egg (beaten)

Method:
Preheat your oven to 180C/160C Fan/350F/Gas mark 4 and have a greaseproofed baking tray to hand.
Roll out the puff pastry until it is around 1/2 cm thick. Cut it into 6 equal squares.

Place the mince and diced vegetables in the centre of each of the pieces of puff pastry leaving a 1cm gap around the edges.

Brush the edges of the pastry with beaten egg and then fold each of the puff pastry pieces over to form triangles.

Pinch the edges of the Cornish pastries to seal them and then place them on the baking tray. Bake them in the oven for 35-45 mins until they are cooked through and then serve.

Spiced Sweet Potato And Feta Wraps (Serves 4)

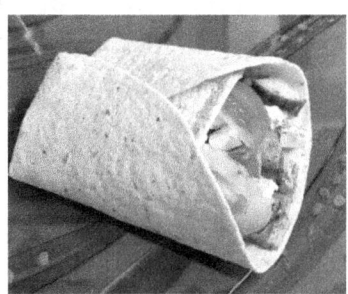

I'm always on the lookout for tasty things to make for my packed lunches, so when I discovered a sweet potato which was languishing in the back of my fridge one evening I decided to make Spiced Sweet Potato and Feta Wraps for lunch the following day with it. The wraps work very well as a light lunch and they make a refreshing change from the usual crumbly gluten-free sandwich fare that most workday lunchtimes are based around. Also, if you fancy this for lunch one day when you're at home you could fold the wraps into parcels and then fry them in a bit of oil until crispy if you'd like to turn them into chimichangas.

Ingredients:

280g sweet potato (peeled and cubed)

160g feta (cubed) (or non-dairy version)

2 tsps oil

1/2 tsp smoked paprika

1/2 tsp ground cumin

2 tsps dried oregano

1/4 tsp dried chilli flakes (optional)

4 gluten-free wraps

Method:

Preheat your oven to 200C/180C Fan/400F/Gas Mark 6 and have a baking tray to hand.

Prepare the sweet potato as directed and place the cubes on a baking tray.

Scatter the oil, herbs and spices on top of the sweet potato and toss them through until they are equally coated.

Bake the sweet potato in the oven for 15 to 20 mins until it is soft and then place the sweet potato inside the wraps along with cubed feta and salad. Serve.

Vegetable Samosas (Makes 8)

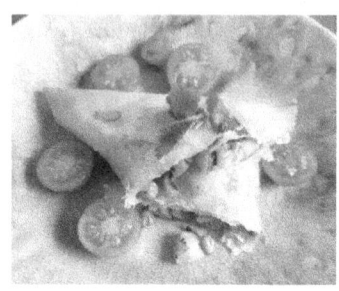

Samosas are traditionally made with shortcrust pastry, but I prefer the flaky crunch that puff pastry provides. Also, as I've said before, I think it's easier to find and buy gluten-free puff pastry. Samosas can be fried or baked, but I prefer baking them because they're healthier and less oil-laden. Although they're traditionally eaten as a starter or a snack to accompany curry I think that they make a brilliant option for lunch and they're delicious when served alongside a fresh salad. Up to three samosas per serving is a low FODMAP portion.

Ingredients:

500g gluten-free puff pastry

1large potato (around 200g) (peeled and diced)

1 carrot (around 80g) (peeled and diced)

1 tbsp. fresh ginger (minced)

40g frozen peas

¼ tsp dried chilli flakes (optional)

1 tbsp. lemon juice

2 tbsps. fresh coriander leaves (chopped)

1 tsp dried ground coriander

½ tsp dried ground cumin

½ tsp garam masala

¼ tsp salt

¼ tsp ground black pepper

1 egg (beaten – to use as egg wash)

Method:
Preheat your oven to 200C/180C Fan/400F/Gas mark 6 and line a flat baking tray with greaseproof paper.
Roll out the puff pastry into a large rectangle and cut it into 8 squares.
Place the diced potato, carrots and peas onto a plate and microwave them until the potato is soft. Put the vegetables into a large bowl and mix the rest of the ingredients into it.
Divide the spiced vegetable mixture between the 8 pieces of pastry leaving a 1cm gap around the edges and brush the edges with egg wash.
Fold one corner of each pasty over to its opposite corner to create a triangle, press the edges down with the tines of a fork and then egg wash the whole pasty before placing them on the greaseproofed baking tray.
Bake them in the oven until the pastry is golden brown and then serve.

Roasted Red Pepper And Tomato Salad (Serves 4)

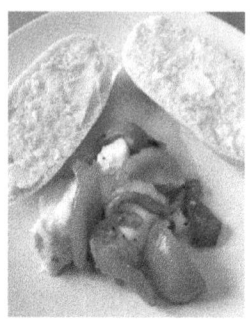

Ingredients:

8 common tomatoes (cut into 6 wedges)

2 red bell peppers (cored and sliced)

4 tbsps. olive oil

4 tsps. red wine vinegar

Salt and pepper to taste

Like most of my cooking, this salad isn't particularly fancy as such, but it makes for a very flavoursome meal. When roasted, the natural sugars found in the red peppers and tomatoes get heightened and take on an almost caramelised sort of flavour.

I like to serve this salad with torn chunks of fresh mozzarella (low FODMAP in servings of up to 40g per portion) and warm gluten-free crusty rolls that have just came straight from the oven and have been generously slathered with real butter.

This salad keeps for a good couple of days in the fridge, so it's also an option to take for packed lunches too. In fact, I often take it to work with some sliced roast chicken on the side or slices of cooked ham and it keeps me going all afternoon.

Method:

Preheat your oven to 200C/180C Fan/400F/Gas Mark 6.

Prepare the vegetables as directed and put them in an ovenproof pan.

Toss them through the olive oil and red wine vinegar.

Add a bit of salt and pepper on top and bake them in the oven for around half an hour until soft.

Serve with fresh mozzarella and crusty rolls.

Sides

Sides

P.56 - Ratatouille

P.57 - Baba Ganoush

P.58 - Roasted Carrot Hummus

P.59 - Blue Cheese Salad Dressing

P.60 - Basil and Walnut Pesto

P.61 - Onion and Garlic Infused Oils

P.62 - Stuffed Potato Skins

P.63 - Sesame Sautéed Broccoli and Bell Pepper

P.64 - Greek Salad

P.65 - Roasted Radishes

P.66 - Crispy Kale

P.67 - Cheese and Chive Baked Baguettes

P.68 - Sage and 'Onion' Stuffing

P.69 - Spiced Red Cabbage

Ratatouille (Serves 4-6)

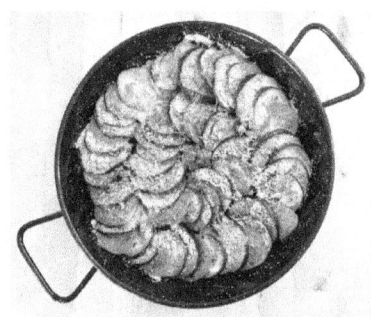

Ratatouille is an excellent side dish to serve with meals, particularly if they're Italian based. However, this ratatouille is substantial enough that if you're vegetarian or vegan it's enough to have as a main meal. This ratatouille is made with courgettes, aubergine and common tomatoes. The vegetables are placed in a casserole dish along with Mediterranean herbs before being drizzled with balsamic glaze and scattered with grated parmesan. This layering ensures that the vegetables become tender and sweet while creating a parmesan crisp on top. It really celebrates summer!

Ingredients:

240g courgettes (thinly sliced)

160g aubergine (thinly sliced)

300g common tomatoes (thinly sliced)

15g capers

60g grated parmesan (or non-dairy)

1 tsp dried oregano

1 tsp dried thyme

1 tbsp balsamic glaze

Ground black pepper

Method:

Preheat your oven to 200C/180C Fan/400F/Gas Mark 6.

Place alternating slices of vegetables in a casserole dish before adding the capers and drizzling the vegetables with balsamic glaze, parmesan and ground black pepper.

Bake in the oven for 30-40 mins until the vegetables are soft and the parmesan is crispy and golden brown. Serve.

Baba Ganoush (Serves 6)

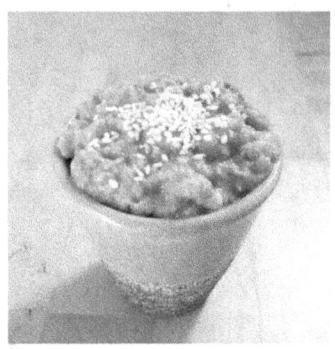

Ingredients:

1 aubergine (no more than 240g prepared weight in total)

1 tbsp garlic-infused oil

1 tbsp peanut butter

1 tbsp lemon juice

1/2 tsp ground cumin (add more to taste)

1/4 tsp dried ground chilli (optional)

2 tbsps fresh chopped parsley

Baba Ganoush is an aubergine dip which originates from Syria and is comprised of roasted, pulped aubergine. It's normally made with tahini, but it's high FODMAP, so I use peanut butter in mine instead and it works brilliantly because it adds a smooth creaminess to the blended aubergine which melds with the lemon juice beautifully.

I like to make my Baba Ganoush with a small amount of cumin and dried chilli just to add a little spiciness and background heat to it, but they are entirely optional steps because the sweet roasted aubergine of the Baba Ganoush is really delicious on its own anyway.

It's a gorgeous dip to accompany warmed flat breads, crackers and vegetable crudités, but it's also really nice on hot toast for breakfast or lunch. However you decide to eat this Baba Ganoush you can be assured that it is light, flavoursome and extremely moreish.

Method:
Preheat your oven to 180C/160 Fan/350F/Gas Mark 5.
Cut the top off the aubergine and then cut the aubergine in half along its length.
Score the flesh of the aubergine in a criss-cross pattern almost all of the way through without breaking the skin and brush the flesh all over with the garlic-infused oil.
Bake the aubergine in the oven for 30-40 mins until the flesh is soft and then leave it to cool.
Scoop the flesh out of the aubergine (discarding the skin) and place it in a bowl and then add all of the rest of the ingredients and mash it all together.
Season to taste and serve.

Roasted Carrot Hummus (Serves 6)

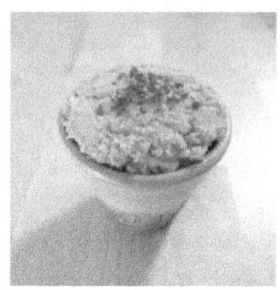

Ingredients:

300g carrots (washed until clean and cut into thick chunks)

2 common tomatoes (cut in half)

1 tbsp vegetable oil

160g tinned chickpeas (drained and well rinsed)

30g peanut butter

1 tbsp lemon juice

1/4 tsp salt

1/4 tsp ground white pepper

I created this roasted carrot hummus for dinner when my vegan step-son came to visit and we all thoroughly enjoyed it. Hummus is traditionally made with chickpeas which are blended with a mixture of spices and tahini to make a smooth, spicy dip which can be served with vegetable crudités, flatbreads, crackers or anything else that takes your fancy. However, chickpeas are high FODMAP, so I incorporate roasted carrots and tomatoes which massively lowers the FODMAP content while adding a huge boost of flavour at the same time.

Carrots are a naturally sweet vegetable, but roasting them in a little bit of oil really increases their inherent sweetness, adding a wonderful caramelised flavour to the hummus. I also like to add a little bit of peanut butter into the roasted carrot hummus because it makes it taste beautifully creamy and provides a gorgeous contrast to the tart, zesty fresh lemon juice which is mixed in. If you like, you can add spices to this roasted carrot hummus too, such as chilli, ground cumin or even smoked paprika.

Method:

Preheat your oven to 200C/180C Fan/400F/Gas mark 6.

Prepare your carrots and tomatoes and put them on a baking tray and toss them in the oil before roasting them until the carrots are soft. (Takes around 30 mins.)

Leave the vegetables to cool. Once they are cold blend all of the ingredients together in a food processor until it forms a thick paste. (You can have your hummus as smooth or chunky as you like.)

Taste for seasoning, adding more if you like, and serve. (I like to add a little dried chopped chilli on top of mine for a bit of a spicy kick.)

Blue Cheese Salad Dressing (Serves 4)

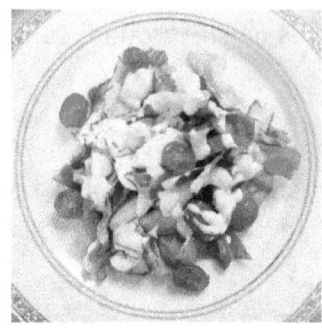

I know that the topic of blue cheese is a divisive one with many people thinking it's repugnant, but when it's used as an ingredient and mixed together with other items it can be a wonderful addition to a meal. Think of anchovies, fish sauce or Worcestershire sauce. On their own they're pretty horrible, but when combined in recipes along with other ingredients they become something special, right?

The first time I put blue cheese in a salad dressing I was really sceptical. Don't get me wrong, I do like blue cheese, but I couldn't imagine how it would work as a salad dressing. However, I'm really pleased to say that my reservations were unfounded because the dressing pairs beautifully with crisp little gem salad leaves, crunchy cubes of cucumber and quartered tomatoes. If you like a bit of blue cheese I'd really encourage you to try this salad dressing. It's rich and creamy while remaining light and refreshing at the same time.

Ingredients:

80g gorgonzola cheese

200g lactose-free natural yoghurt

20g mayonnaise

1 tbsp. lemon juice

½ tsp ground black pepper

3 tbsps. fresh chives (finely chopped)

Method:

Simply mix all of the ingredients together until a smooth creamy sauce is formed. Serve.

Basil And Pine Nut Pesto (Serves 5)

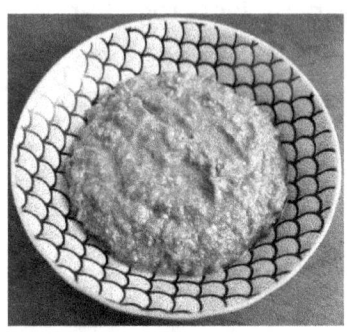

It's a great idea to have a pesto recipe on hand at all times because aside from being a tasty alternative to mayonnaise in sandwiches, it's also a great standby sauce that brings pasta alive. In the summer I tend to grow basil myself from seed and it grows like wildfire, so to use it up (although it's never really a hardship) I always have a pot of pesto on the go in the fridge.

I like my pesto to be quite thick and robust, but you can make yours looser if you like by adding more olive oil to the mix. However, do remember that although fats are FODMAP free they can have an impact on your gut motility, so exercise caution. In total this recipe makes 5 low FODMAP portions of pesto.

Ingredients:

50g fresh basil leaves

50g pine nuts

75ml mild olive oil (or more if you want a looser pesto)

30g grated parmesan (or non-dairy version)

1/4 tsp ground black pepper

1/4 tsp salt (or more, to suit your own taste)

Method:

Put all of the ingredients into a NutriBullet, blender or food processor and blend until either smooth or slightly chunky. Serve.

Onion And Garlic Infused Oils

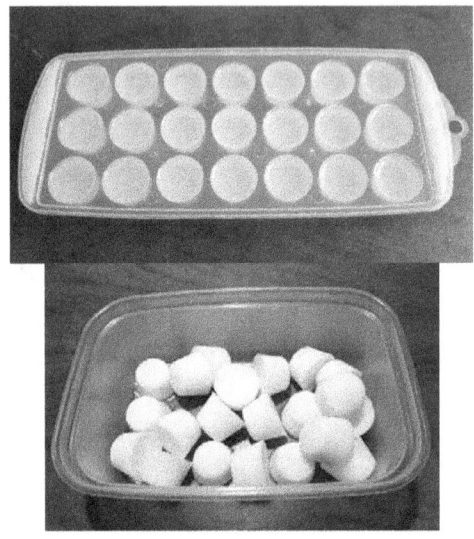

A lot of people who begin the low FODMAP diet aren't aware that they can still enjoy the flavours of onion and garlic in their cooking by using onion and garlic-infused oils due to the fact that the FODMAPs found in onion and garlic are only soluble in water. In other words they aren't absorbed into oil, but their unique flavours are.

You can, of course, buy onion and garlic infused oils from supermarkets, but they tend to be quite pricy where I live, so I find it much cheaper to make them myself. For safety reasons I don't like the idea of keeping infused oils in the cupboard or fridge just in case bacteria develops, so I pour my oil into silicone ice-cube trays and freeze them. That way I can just pop a cube out as and when I need them.

I make mine quite strong, so that I don't need to use much oil in my cooking, but feel free to lower the amount of onion and garlic you use to suit your own taste.

Ingredients for the Garlic Oil:

500ml oil

8 cloves of garlic (thinly sliced)

Ingredients for the Onion Oil:

500ml oil

2 onions (thickly sliced)

Method:
Follow this method to make both oils.

Put the oil in a large saucepan over a low heat until it is warm to the touch and then add the onion or garlic slices. Take the pan off the heat and then leave it to infuse for 2-3 hours.

After this time, place a sieve over a large jug and drain the oil through the sieve to remove all of the onion or garlic pieces.

Pour the oil into silicone ice-cube trays and then lie them flat in your freezer and freeze them until required.

Stuffed Potato Skins (Serves 2-4)

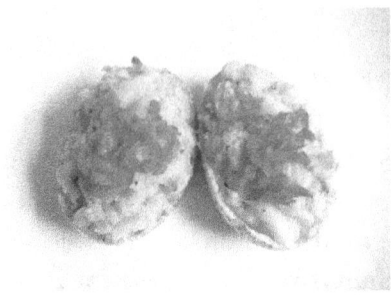

Stuffed potato skins are one of those delicious side dishes that you just can't resist ordering in restaurants, but they're actually really easy to make at home too. Loaded with melting cheddar cheese and chunks of smoked bacon they're a brilliant addition to any meal, although they can also make for a very substantial and tasty main meal on their own too.

I tend to stick with making mine with the classic combination of cheddar and bacon, but you can make them vegetarian or vegan by using non-dairy cheese and pairing it with diced bell peppers and oyster mushrooms (up to 70g per person). I also like to sprinkle a little bit of chopped fresh chilli on top, but that step's entirely optional.

Ingredients:

2 large baking potatoes

80g grated cheddar cheese or mozzarella (or non-dairy version)

4 rashers of smoked bacon (finely chopped)

2 tbsps of chopped chives

1/4 tsp ground black pepper

Chopped fresh chilli (optional)

Method:

Bake the 2 potatoes whole for 45-60 mins until they are soft in the middle.

Cut the potatoes in half lengthwise and scoop out the flesh (trying not to damage the skins) and put the flesh in a bowl.

Add the grated cheese, bacon, pepper and chives to the potato in the bowl and mash it all together.

Stuff the potato skins with the potato mixture and bake them in the oven for another 25-30 mins. Serve.

Sesame Sautéed Broccoli And Red Pepper (Serves 2)

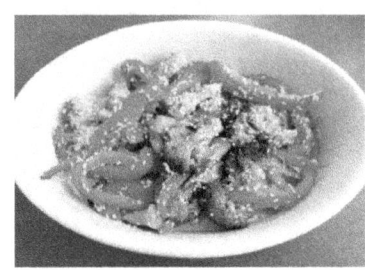

I used to always think that I preferred Indian flavours over Asian ones until I discovered the wonder ingredient which is sesame oil. It's such a versatile oil which adds a delicious toasted, nutty flavour to any Asian meal and really elevates the taste of the whole dish.

This recipe celebrates the flavour of sesame through its use of sesame oil and sesame seeds, both of which pair beautifully with the freshness of broccoli florets and the sweetness of sliced red bell peppers.

This is an ideal side dish to make if you're looking for something to bulk out an Asian-inspired meal, but it's also delicious enough to make as a quick vegetarian or vegan snack or even as a vegetable-filled light lunch. In fact, if you add some cooked rice and a little soy sauce mixed with a bit of minced ginger you've got a ready-made packed lunch waiting to happen!

Ingredients:

100g whole broccoli florets

1 tbsp. sesame oil

1 tbsp. sesame seeds

1 red bell pepper (deseeded and thinly sliced)

Salt and pepper

Method:

Steam or boil your broccoli until it is tender and then drain it well.

Heat the sesame oil in a large frying pan over a medium heat and once it's hot add the vegetables and sesame seeds.

Cook until the red pepper is soft enough to your liking and then season and serve.

Greek Salad (Serves 1 As A Main Or 2 As A Side)

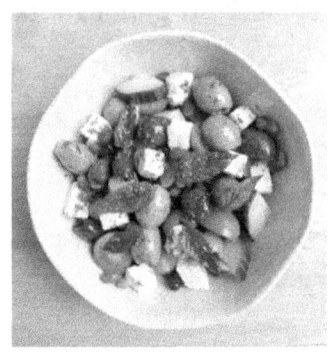

Ingredients:

14 black and green olives

1/4 of a cucumber (diced)

40g cubed feta cheese (or non-dairy version)

1 common tomato (thinly sliced into wedges)

1 tsp olive oil

1/2 tsp red wine vinegar

1/2 tsp dried oregano

2 tbsps pomegranate seeds

8 fresh mint leaves

Greek salad is an incredible salad to serve as a side dish, but because it contains cubed feta cheese, mixed olives and chunks of fresh cucumber it's substantial enough to serve as a main meal for lunch too. It's also seriously FODMAP-friendly because as long as you keep to the recommended amount of feta and pomegranate seeds per portion it's very low FODMAP.

In fact, if you're highly intolerant to fructose you can easily leave the pomegranate seeds out without it massively affecting the overall taste of the Greek salad. And, of course, if you're lactose intolerant or allergic to dairy you can replace the feta cheese with a dairy-free version if you like.

Taking into consideration that this Greek salad is 'just' a salad, it's actually very filling and satisfying, its individual components coming together to blend into a harmonious bowlful of very refreshing ingredients.

This Greek salad sees mixed black and green olives paired with crisp cubes of cucumber, sweet, tangy tomato wedges and salty, creamy feta cheese, all of which is tossed in a fresh, tart vinaigrette made from olive oil, red wine vinegar and oregano. It's a timeless salad which you will welcome at any time of the day.

Method:

Keep the pomegranate seeds and mint leaves to one side and then prepare the rest of the ingredients as directed and place them in a bowl.

Mix the olive oil and red wine vinegar with the oregano and drizzle it over the ingredients in the bowl.

Decorate with the pomegranate seeds and mint leaves and then serve.

Roasted Radishes (Serves 4)

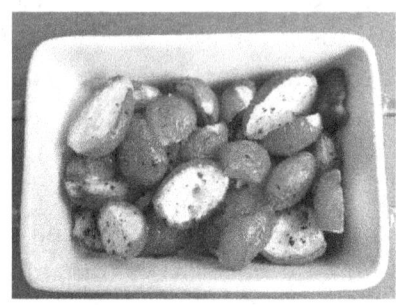

Radishes are a vegetable which is completely free of FODMAPs, so if you've a taste for them it makes sense to embrace them as part of your low FODMAP diet. As a result of them being FODMAP-free I always grow radishes in the greenhouse to eat as they are or to add to salads, but last year I planted too many at once and it resulted in me having quite a glut of radishes all at once. (I'm still very much a gardening novice.) That's when this recipe was born.

Radishes might not seem like the normal type of vegetable that you would roast, but they're so tasty! Upon roasting they develop a natural sweetness and their texture changes from a crisp apple-like crunch to a softer, more delicate bite. Their peppery taste also means you can pair them with other flavours, such as sprigs of fresh thyme or rosemary, or you can add strips of smoked bacon to the pan before you roast them. If you've never tried roasted radishes before then I truly implore you to give them a go. You won't be disappointed!

Ingredients:

200g halved radishes

1 tbsp. vegetable oil

Salt and pepper

Method:

Preheat your oven to 200C/180C Fan/400F/Gas mark 6.

Top and tail the radishes before halving them and coating them in the oil and scattering salt and pepper over them. (If you're roasting them with fresh herbs or bacon add them at this point.) Roast them in the oven for 20-25 mins and then serve.

Crispy Kale (Serves 2)

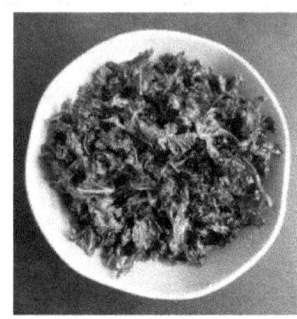

Ingredients:

140g fresh chopped kale (with the hard stalks removed)

2 tbsps. vegetable oil

¼ tsp salt & ¼ tsp ground pepper

1 tsp white sugar

When the whole 'kale fad' began I was very sceptical as to how tasty it would actually be because I'm sure many of us were brought up on steamed greens and know just how utterly bland they can be.

However, crispy kale – kale that's been tossed in oil and seasoning and then toasted in the oven until crunchy- is a different thing altogether!

Cooking the kale in this manner brings out the naturally nutty flavour of the fresh kale while infusing it with the sweet and salty taste of good seasoning. I think that it tastes just like the crispy seaweed side dish you can buy from Asian restaurants!

As a result, we have this crispy kale quite frequently because it's a great way to incorporate kale into our diets without it feeling like a trial. Give it a go and see what you think!

Method:

Preheat your oven to 200C/180C Fan/400F/Gas mark 6 and have a large baking tray to hand.

Remove the hard kale stalks then put the kale into a large bowl and mix the oil, salt, pepper and sugar through it with your hands until all of the kale is coated with the oil.

Spread it out evenly on the baking tray and bake it for 4-5 mins before mixing it all up and spreading it out again and baking it again.

 (This ensures that all of the kale gets steadily toasted evenly, but watch out because it can burn easily!)

Once the kale is golden brown and crisp remove it from the oven and serve it immediately.

Cheese And Chive Baked Baguettes (Serves 2-4)

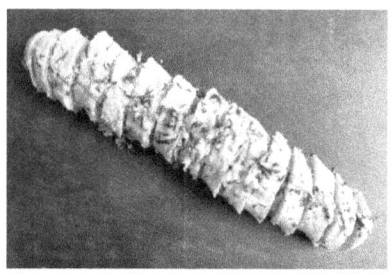

I'm always on the look-out for low FODMAP side dishes and these cheese and chive baked baguettes are a brilliant example because they can be paired with loads of main meals and can feed a lot of people too. They're really good served with Italian meals like lasagne or spaghetti bolognese, but we've even had them with things like a late breakfast/brunch Shakshuka.

Ingredients:

1 gluten-free part-baked baguette

2 tbsps of chopped fresh chives

80g of lactose-free cheddar cheese or mozzarella (or a non-dairy version)

1/2 tsp ground black pepper

Method:

Preheat your oven to 200C/180C Fan/400F/Gas mark 6.

Mix the grated cheese, chives and black pepper together in a bowl.

Place the baguette on a baking tray and cut slices into the baguette and stuff them with the cheese and chive mixture.

Bake the baguette in the oven until the cheese has all melted. Serve alongside your chosen meal.

Sage And 'Onion' Stuffing (Serves 4-8)

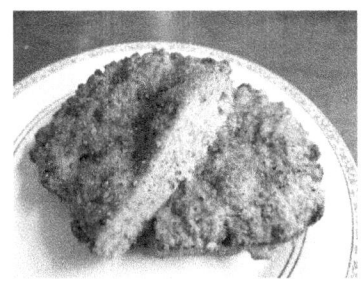

Everyone knows that a roast chicken dinner is not complete without tasty sage and onion stuffing served on the side, but due to the constraints of the low FODMAP diet most sage and onion stuffing mixes are unsuitable due to the inclusion of onion in the mix. However, that's where this recipe comes in.

I've written before about the low FODMAP wonder that is asafoetida spice and its oniony-flavoured properties and it's put to good use here. Asafoetida is completely low FODMAP and is a great substitute for onion when a recipe demands onion flavours. The asafoetida works brilliantly with the dried sage to produce a well-seasoned and herby pork stuffing which absolutely sings with flavour.

Some people would use an egg to bind the stuffing, but I don't think it's necessary because the sausage meat will have fat in it which will help to firm it up.

Ingredients:

450g gluten-free pork sausage meat

130g gluten-free breadcrumbs

2 tsps. dried sage

2 tbsps. dried parsley

½ tsp asafoetida powder

2 tbsps. dried chives

½ tsp ground black pepper

Method:

Preheat your oven to 200C/180C Fan/400F/Gas Mark 6.

Simply mix all of the ingredients together in a mixing bowl and once it's combined flatten it into a casserole dish.

Bake it in the oven for 25-30 mins until it is cooked through and golden brown.

Serve.

Spiced Red Cabbage (Serves 10-14)

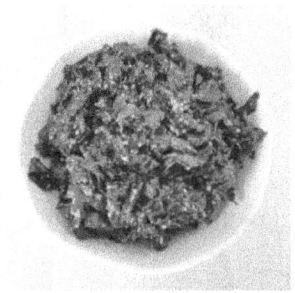

Ingredients:

500g red cabbage (quartered, cored and shredded)

100g brown sugar

150ml red wine vinegar

The zest and juice of 1 orange

1 tbsp. oil

1 tbsp. mustard seeds

1 star anise

½ tsp asafoetida powder

¼ of a freshly grated nutmeg

15g fresh minced ginger

1 tsp ground allspice

The first time I ate spiced red cabbage was when it was served alongside a meal I was having in a restaurant around Christmastime. At first, upon tasting it, I didn't really understand why such a sweet-tasting accompaniment would be served alongside meat, but once my palate acclimatised I realised that the spiced red cabbage just worked as a tasty condiment type of side dish to complement the roast chicken it came with.

It can be hard (dare I even say almost impossible?) to find low FODMAP chutneys and relishes, so this recipe has been a welcome addition to my meals. It's a brilliant chutney substitute and it works really well with a wide range of dishes. (Think of it served alongside meals like roast chicken or beef, sausages, and even in a cheese sandwich.)

Due to its versatility I tend to cook a big batch of it at a time and keep some of it in the fridge to use within a week and I freeze the rest of it in small portions to defrost as and when I need it. It's just a great low FODMAP side option.

Method:

Heat the oil in a large saucepan over a medium heat and add the ginger, cabbage, spices and the zest and juice of the orange.

Cook until the cabbage is soft.

Add the sugar and red wine vinegar to the pan and cook for 15-20 mins until the liquid has reduced down to a sticky glaze.

Serve.

Part 2

Introduction

The FODMAP diet has been developed and tested in practice by scientists at Monash University in Melbourne. At the Monash University of Melbourne, Professor Peter Gibson and Susan Shepherd have developed the FODMAP diet. Dr. Sue Shepherd is an Advanced Accredited Practicing Dietitian and an Advanced Accredited Nutritionist. She specializes in the treatment of food intolerances. Peter Gibson is professor and director of Gastroenterology at The Alfred and Monash University in Australia, and formerly professor of Medicine and Head of the Eastern Health Clinical School. The FODMAP-restricted diet is a diet from which several products are omitted for at least 2-6 weeks. Think of some vegetables, fruits, wheat and dairy products.

Fodmap Research

There is a growing number of scientific studies from around the world to support the fact that reducing FODMAPs in the diet can help reduce symptoms in people with irritable bowel syndrome (PDS) or other functional bowel complaints (FGA). The FODMAP diet is not a fad diet: the diet is supported by scientific evidence, and its use is increasing internationally. For example, a scientific study conducted in the UK proved that the low FODMAP diet is beneficial in alleviating symptoms (76% of participants achieved symptom control). A study was recently conducted at Martini Hospital in Groningen with 30 patients with IBS who had been selected by their doctor. The group had to follow the diet for 6-8 weeks strictly. Subsequently, high FODMAP products were reintroduced into the diet. The patients received guidance from the dietitians from the hospital. Of the 30 patients, no fewer than 73% had fewer complaints by following the diet. After reintroduction, hypersensitivity to lactose, polyols (carbohydrates found in, for example, cabbages, legumes, and sweeteners) and fructans (carbohydrates in fruit and honey) were found. Two patients dropped out prematurely because the diet blocked them. The researchers are hopeful that the FODMAP diet is an effective treatment for most people with irritable bowel syndrome, also because it appears from research in other countries. Thus, there are more and more investigations.

What are fodmaps
FODMAPs are nutrients (molecules) that can cause complaints such as gas formation and abdominal pain. The nutrients are short-chain carbohydrates and related alcohols: oligosaccharides of fructose (fructans) and galactose (galactans), disaccharides (lactose), monosaccharide (fructose), and sugar alcohols (polyols) such as sorbitol, mannitol, xylitol and maltitol. These nutrients are poorly or not absorbed in the small intestine and end up in the large intestine.

Spastic intestine, IBS, intestinal complaints
Everyone poorly absorbs FODMAP carbohydrates. All FODMAPs that are not absorbed in the small intestine goes to the large intestine. There the carbohydrates are quickly fermented or converted by the intestinal bacteria that are present there. This results in the production of substances and gases, causing the intestine to swell. In people with sensitive intestines (spastic

intestine, IBS) this gives a bloated feeling and flatulence. These carbohydrates can also attract moisture in the intestine, causing the intestine to swell. Because of the pressure, you get a bloated stomach and pain. Examples of these carbohydrates are lactose (milk sugar), fructose (fruit sugar), and carbohydrates from wheat, cabbage, and beans.

Prevalence: how many people have an irritable bowel?

The Irritable Bowel Syndrome (PDS) occurs in the general Dutch population (measured with self-reporting) in 15 to 20% of women and 5 to 20% of men. The incidence in general practice (CMR) for the period 1998 to 2006 is 2 to 3 per 1000 per year for men and 6 to 7 per 1000 per year for women. The prevalence is 4 per 1000 for men and 10 per 1000 for women. Internationally, PDS has an estimated prevalence of 14 to 24% in women and 5 to 19%. This means that almost 2 million Dutch people have PD complaints! The FODMAP diet works with a large proportion of people with IBS. According to studies, the evidence is between 50 and 85%. If you calculated this, 1 million Dutch people would benefit from the FODMAP diet!

FODMAPs are naturally found in foods that we eat every day and form the basis for a healthy diet.

FODMAP is an abbreviation for:

F - Fermentable

O - Oligosaccharides (fructans and galactans).

D - Disaccharides (lactose).

These are found in milk products.

M - Monosaccharaides (fructose).

These are found in fruits and vegetables.

A - And

P - Polyols (sugar alcohols).

These are found in sweeteners, fruits, and vegetables.

FODMAPs are small molecules (carbohydrates) that are poorly or not absorbed in the small intestine and end up in the large intestine. There are many bacteria in the colon. These bacteria then ferment (= eat) the FODMAPs quickly and in vast quantities. This releases gas, causing symptoms such as bloating and flatulence. Symptoms such as diarrhea or disturbed bowel movements arise because more fluid is attracted to the small and large intestines. By restricting products with many FODMAPs in the diet, fewer of these molecules enter the colon. Not everyone is equally sensitive. In practice, small amounts of FODMAPs give no complaints.

The Different Fodmaps
The different FODMAPs are discussed here one by one.

For each group, you will find a link to a list of foods that are FODMAP-poor or FODMAP-rich.

The information about the content of FODMAPs comes mostly from the Monash University in Melbourne. You may miss products on the lists. For example, typical Dutch products that they do not know in Australia or that have not been analyzed. Ask your dietician for more information.

Apps: The Monash University Low FODMAP Diet app (for Android and iPhone) can be a useful tool.

NB: There are several apps available for the low FODMAP diet. We have not checked this for reliability.

- **Oligosaccharides**

Of the oligosaccharides, fructans, and Galatians give the most complaints.

- **Fructans**

The primary sources of fructans are wheat products (bread, cereals, and pasta) and some vegetables, such as onions. Other sources of fructans are inulin and fructooligosaccharides (also known as oligofructose and FOS), which have been added as prebiotics to individual lean yogurts and milk drinks and to some dietary fiber preparations. The food industry uses inulin as a product improver in, for example, skimmed milk products. No one can digest fructans. Fructans are probably the leading causes of IBS symptoms, probably because most people eat a lot of them. They are found in many different foods and large quantities in our food supply. We have made a list of low fructan and fructan luxurious products.

- **Galactans**

Galactans or galactooligosaccharides (GOS) are most commonly found in food in the form of raffinose and stachyose. They are found in legumes such as kidney beans, lentils, and chickpeas. Like fructans, galactans cannot be digested or absorbed by anyone and can cause many complaints in people with IBS.

We have made a list of low- galactan and galactan-rich products.

- **Disaccharides**

Only one disaccharide can behave as a FODMAP in food: lactose.

- **Lactose**

Lactose occurs naturally in mammalian milk, including cow's milk, sheep's milk, and goat's milk. Lactose is split in the small intestine by the enzyme lactase, after which it can be absorbed. Lactase is located in the wall of the small intestine. In the case of a deficiency of this enzyme, lactose malabsorption occurs, and complaints that occur with this are called lactose intolerance. The number of lactase enzymes can differ per person, depending on factors such as ethnicity (people of Asian origin often make little lactase) and the presence of specific intestinal disorders. A lactose-restricted diet is not a dairy-free diet: we have made a list of low- lactose and lactose-rich products.

- **Monosaccharides**

The only important monosaccharide that can act as a FODMAP in food is fructose.

- **Fructose**

Fructose, also known as fruit sugar, is found in large quantities in various foods, especially in certain fruits and honey. It is also added to many food products as a sweetener or to improve appearance or texture. An excess of fructose can cause PDS symptoms in some people, which we call fructose intolerance. They do not have to avoid fructose (or fruit) altogether. As long as the fructose is in balance with glucose or food contains more glucose than fructose, small amounts can be eaten at a time without inducing PDS symptoms.

It is better to take a small portion of the suitable types of fruit as a snack a few times a day than in one goes. We have made a list of low- fructose and fructose-rich products.

- **Polyols**

Polyols are carbohydrates that are poorly absorbed by many people. Polyols have names ending with 'ol' and include, among others, sorbitol, mannitol, maltitol, and xylitol. They occur naturally in some fruits, especially stone fruits, and vegetables. They are often used in the food industry as humectants (substances that retain moisture) and artificial sweeteners - especially in 'sugar-free' chewing gum, peppermint, and sweets. When used as an artificial sweetener, polyols can be recognized by their E numbers - sorbitol (E420), mannitol (E421), maltitol (E965), xylitol (E967). The package also states: "Excessive use can have a laxative effect". The added substance isomalt can have the same effect. Low polyol and luxurious polyol products.

Overview of fodmap-poor and fodmap-rich foods

Here is a list of FODMAP poor and FODMAP luxurious products.

Read labels

Much information about a product can be found on the label. Manufacturers are, in fact, obliged to report ingredients on their products. All ingredients must be listed in descending order of weight, except mixtures of fruit and vegetables. So the sooner an ingredient is mentioned, the more of that ingredient is in the product. Eating a small amount of FODMAP will not hurt. A product can change its composition over time, so keep checking the labels regularly.

Ingredients that should be avoided are not always natural to recognize on the label. The list below can help with this.

FODMAPs   Ingredients

Fructan   Inulin

FOS   Oligofructose

Fructose, fructose syrup, glucose-fructose syrup, and fructose corn syrup

Lactose, buttermilk, milk constituents, milk powder, and whey

Polyols   Isomalt, maltitol, mannitol, sorbitol and xylitol (E numbers - sorbitol (E420), mannitol (E421), maltitol (E965), xylitol (E967))

How Do Fodmaps Cause Symptoms Of Ibs?

All FODMAPs have the same four properties:

1. FODMAPs are poorly absorbed in the small intestine.

This means that many of these FODMAP- molecules are not absorbed in the small intestine and instead end up undigested in the large intestine. The reason for this is that they cannot be broken down by the intestine into smaller molecules or that the mechanism is too slow to be able to absorb all molecules during the passage through the small intestine (in the case of fructose). How well we can digest and absorb some FODMAPs varies from person to person - fructose absorption is slow for everyone. However, for some people very slowly, some people (especially with dark skin color) do not produce enough enzymes (lactase) to produce lactose to break down, and also, the ability to absorb polyols varies from person to person. Since nobody can digest fructans and galactans (these are found in wheat, for example),

Carbohydrates that can be easily digested, such as sucrose (table sugar) or glucose, give no complaints.

2. FODMAPs are small molecules that can be present in our diet in a large amount.

When a large amount of small molecules is in the small intestine, they will attract water through the osmotic effect. Extra fluid in the digestive tract can cause diarrhea, increase pain through volume increase, and affect muscle movements in the gut.

3. FODMAPs are food for the bacteria that naturally live in the colon.

If molecules are not taken up in the small intestine, they will end up in the large intestine. The colon contains innumerable bacteria by nature. The bacteria that live there feed on these molecules and break them down quickly, releasing the gases hydrogen, carbon dioxide, and methane. You call this fermentation. This gas production can lead to flatulence, flatulence, feeling uncomfortable, or pain in the abdomen. The pain complaints are probably caused by a pressure increase in the sensitive intestine of PDS patients.

Also, gas production (methane gas) can probably delay the movement of food residues through the colon in some people and thus contribute to blockage. How fast the molecules are fermented depends on the length of their sugar chain: small molecules such as oligosaccharides and sugars are fermented very quickly compared to dietary fibers.

4. The effect is cumulative

A single meal usually contains multiple types of FODMAPs. Because they all cause complaints of the intestine in the same way once they reach the lower part of the small intestine and colon, their effects are cumulative. This means that the effects of all different FODMAPs must be added together. The complaints, therefore, depend on the total of FODMAPs per meal that is eaten (or drunk) and not on the amount of FODMAPs of each type. When someone who cannot digest both lactose and fructose poorly, eats a meal that contains a little of all FODMAPs (lactose, fructans, polyols, galactans, fructose), then the effect on the intestines will be 1 + 1 + 1 + 1 + 1 = 5 times greater than if he or she had eaten or drunk the same amount of only one of this FODMAPs. Therefore, the total amount of FODMAPs in the meals must be assessed when adjusting the diet.

The amount of gas and liquid in the intestines can be reduced by reducing the amount of FODMAPs in the diet with the FODMAP-restricted diet and by eating smaller portions more spread throughout the day.

Why Don't We All Suffer From Pds?
We all eat FODMAPs and produce gas, so why does one person receive PDS and the other not? There are five possible reasons for this:

1. How much gas we produce. This depends on the types of bacteria that live in the intestines and how they process the gas. Each person has a different combination of bacteria in his / her intestines, and some bacteria are more active fermenters (gas formers) than others.
2. The visceral sense of the intestines. Some people's intestines are more sensitive than others. The feeling of a bloated belly depends on the 'adjustment' of our nervous system of the intestine: how much the belly is set up before we start to feel uncomfortable. Only people with a sensitive gut will get complaints after taking too many FODMAPs.
3. How well the intestine can remove gas after it has been formed. When much gas is produced, this usually stimulates the digestive tract to rapidly transport the gas through the intestines until it is emitted as the wind. In some people with IBS, however, the gas remains in the intestines, where it causes a higher degree of abdominal distension.
4. How well the intestines respond to swelling. The abdominal muscles usually contract automatically when the intestines

are set up so that our abdomen does not protrude. When the intestines are set up, the diaphragm (a large muscle located under the lungs) usually relaxes, creating more room in the abdomen for the intestines. However, in some people with IBS, these reflex reactions are feeble. With them, intestinal distension can lead to contraction and therefore flattening of the diaphragm, which makes the abdomen more forward and (female) patients appear pregnant. This also gives a more significant inconvenience.
5. Our awareness of signals from the intestines and how we deal with these signals. Under different circumstances, we deal with signals from the intestines differently. Our perceptions are influenced by stress and what happens in our lives. The intestines can be experienced as more sensitive to stress and fatigue. This is also part of the functioning of the 'brain-intestinal axis.'

To Investigate
There is a growing number of scientific studies from around the world to support the fact that reducing FODMAPs in the diet can help reduce symptoms in people with irritable bowel syndrome (PDS) or other functional bowel complaints (FGA). The FODMAP diet is not a fad diet: the diet is supported by scientific evidence, and its use is increasing internationally. For example, a scientific study conducted in the UK proved that the low FODMAP diet is beneficial in alleviating symptoms (76% of participants achieved symptom control). The Martini Hospital in Groningen conducted a study in 2014 with 30 patients with IBS who were selected by their doctors. The group had to follow the diet for 6-8 weeks strictly. Subsequently, high FODMAP products were reintroduced into the diet. The patients received guidance from the dietitians from the hospital. Of the 30 patients, no fewer than 73% had fewer complaints by following the diet. After reintroduction, hypersensitivity to lactose, polyols (carbohydrates found in, for example, cabbages, legumes, and sweeteners) and fructans (carbohydrates in fruit and honey)

were found. Two patients dropped out prematurely because the diet blocked them. The researchers are hopeful that the FODMAP diet is an effective treatment for most people with irritable bowel syndrome, also because it appears from research in other countries.

Intestinal Complaints
Do you also suffer from your intestines and the feeling that nutrition can be a cause? If so, it can be useful to investigate which substances or food are responsible for this. Many people with intestinal complaints suffer from flatulence or bloating, often caused by too many gasses in the intestines. Gases are produced from colon bacteria by feeding on unabsorbed molecules. This process is called fermentation.

Our diet consists of fats, proteins, carbohydrates, vitamins, and minerals. Many carbohydrates such as dietary fiber are poorly digested and not absorbed in the small intestine. Insoluble dietary fiber cannot be fermented (eaten) by bacteria in the gut, while soluble fiber is fermented by gut bacteria. Some single short-chain sugars (oligosaccharides) and sugar alcohols are also indigestible and/or cannot be absorbed by the gut, but are broken down by the gut bacteria into gases.

Do you also suffer from gases and flatulence? Try to eat fewer carbohydrates; often the complaints will also improve. To keep getting fewer complaints, it is useful to find out which carbohydrates give you complaints.

The short-chain sugars/carbohydrates that many people with intestinal complaints suffer from are fermented by the intestinal bacteria (the fast food for the bacteria). These short-chain sugars are called the FODMAPs. In addition to gases and flatulence, FODMAPs can also cause diarrhea, pain, cramps, and constipation.

Everyone poorly absorbs FODMAP carbohydrates. All FODMAPs that are not absorbed in the small intestine goes to the large intestine. There the carbohydrates are quickly fermented or converted by the intestinal bacteria that are present there. This results in the production of substances and gases, causing the intestine to swell. In people with sensitive intestines (spastic gut, PDS) this gives a bloated feeling and flatulence. These carbohydrates can also attract moisture in the intestine, causing the intestine to swell. Because of the pressure, you get a bloated stomach and pain. Examples of these carbohydrates are lactose (milk sugar), fructose (fruit sugar), and carbohydrates from wheat, cabbage, and beans.

Follow the fodmap diet
If you decide to follow the fodmap diet, it must be sure that your symptoms are based on IBS and not on another disease. That is why we advise you to consult your doctor before starting the diet.

The fodmap diet consists of 2 phases: elimination and reintroduction

The low FODMAP diet consists of 2 parts: the **elimination diet** followed by **reintroduction** to find out what causes the symptoms. The guidelines recommend a diet that lasts for several weeks to substantially reduce the intake of foods with high FODMAPs. In the diet, all these carbohydrates are initially omitted for about four weeks from the diet. That is a pretty strict diet, so calling in a dietician for guidance is not a superfluous luxury. Many people experience a great deal of relief from their complaints in this so-called 'elimination period.' In the following weeks, a group of carbohydrates is always allowed into the diet. For example, fructose (apples, mango, honey) or lactose (milk, yogurt). When the complaints come back, it is clear what the culprits are. Then you return to the essential diet and try a different carbohydrate after a few days. Ultimately, you have a tailor-made diet, without the carbohydrates that give you complaints. You can continue to follow that diet to prevent complaints. It is different per person how much FODMAP intake can be tolerated before symptoms are caused. Reintroduction of FODMAPs is an essential part of the process. It is recommended to follow the diet under the guidance of a dietitian, preferably a specialist in gastrointestinal nutrition. It is different per person how much FODMAP intake can be tolerated before symptoms are caused. Reintroduction of FODMAPs is an essential part of the process. It is recommended to follow the diet under the guidance of a dietitian, preferably a specialist in gastrointestinal nutrition. It is different per person how much FODMAP intake can be tolerated before symptoms are caused. Reintroduction of FODMAPs is an essential part of the process. It is recommended to follow the diet under the guidance of a dietitian, preferably a specialist in gastrointestinal nutrition.

Dietician guidance

The FODMAP diet is not simple. However, the diet is new and not yet known to all dietitians and general practitioners. It can, therefore, be challenging to find a dietitian who is familiar with this diet. Before the 1st phase (elimination phase), the dietitian will advise which foods rich in FODMAPs should be avoided. After this strict low FODMAP restriction, people who follow the diet will go to the dietician again. The dietitian:

a) Assesses how well you respond to dietary restrictions, and

b) Discusses your tolerance level

c) Helps with sufficient variation in your diet

d) helps to prevent you from not getting any nutritional deficiencies (in the long term)

e) Helps when reading labels and how to deal with parties and eating out.

Low-fodmap diet during the festive periods.

Those who follow the low-FODMAP diet often have difficulties with special occasions such as holidays and birthday parties. People are afraid that "mistakes" will be made.

It is essential to know that with the low FODMAP diet, there is intolerance and no allergy. This means that you can tolerate certain foods in specific quantities. The problem with party menus is that many ingredients are mixed in small quantities and that menu are often accompanied by a large consumption of alcohol.

A few tips to get through the holidays without any problems:

Are you a host or hostess yourself? Then you cook a FODMAP menu yourself. Do we bet that no guest will notice anything?

Are you going to eat with friends or family? Inform the host or hostess that you need to make sure nutritional adjustments. If you feel that they have problems adjusting certain things, then propose to bring something yourself, e.g. make the soup yourself or prepare a dessert.

If you go to a restaurant, inform the restaurant well in advance that you are not allowed to eat all the foods and whether they can propose alternatives.

Suggest alternatives yourself, because not every chef is familiar with the FODMAP poor diet.

Tips Per Menu

APERITIF

One glass of dry (sparkling) white wine, cava, prosecco, champagne is allowed, but there are many non-alcoholic alternatives:

- Aperitif with cranberry juice and spray water
- Spray water with lime or lemon
- Infusion of cucumber and lemon

- Spray water with ginger or ginger syrup infusion (check the label for fructose!)

SNACKS WITH THE APERITIF
- Toasts are replaced by crackers based on buckwheat, quinoa.
- Break the crackers into pieces and serve with a tapenade of green or black olives.
- Salty chips.
- Cover crackers with an egg with caviar or fake caviar
- Siege crackers with smoked fish (salmon, halibut, trout) and arugula
- Serve raw vegetables: cut carrots into strips, place cocktail tomatoes in a pot, arrange chicory leaves on a saucer. Serve with a dipping sauce (mayonnaise or cocktail sauce that you make yourself by adding mayonnaise with some tomato puree).
- Skewer with cucumber and hard cheese or cherry tomato and mozzarella.
- Make mini quiches based on rice sheets and use artichoke hearts for the filling.

Be careful with wraps, which often contain polyols (eg glycerol or E422) that can cause problems.

SOUP
- If you make soup, omit onion and garlic.
- Purchased soups will usually contain onion and garlic; the ingredients can be found on the ingredient list.
- Mixed soup vegetables usually contain onion. Do you like to buy pre-sliced soup vegetables? Then choose a non-mixed variety, e.g. celeriac or broccoli florets (in the freezer compartment).
- You can use the green part of spring onion and wild garlic. The green part of the leeks is limited in use (80 grams per portion).

- Be careful with bouillon cubes, but use other flavorings: cook some sprigs of fresh thyme with it or add flavor with fresh herbs (watercress, parsley).
- Use your cream to finish the soup: replace the classic cream with soy cream, rice cream, oat cream, or another vegetable alternative.

MAIN DISHES

- Choose vegetables from the allowed list. Check the method of preparation: without adding sauce, stock cubes, or a mix of vegetable herbs. Best are stewed or steamed vegetables, seasoned with salt and pepper, and fresh herbs.
- Meat, poultry, and fish are not a problem in principle but avoid marinated and breaded preparations.
- Be careful with game stews, stew meat, hare ragout: these dishes contain onion and garlic.
- Replace wheat pasta with buckwheat pasta, rice noodles, or rice-based pasta. There are plenty of tasty alternatives to wheat pasta.
- Ask to serve the sauce separately.

DESSERT

- Sorbet
- Soy ice cream
- Coconut ice cream
- Merengue: based on whipped egg whites and sugar. You can eat this pure or use it as a pie crust, and you can invest with fresh fruit (permitted varieties).
- Fruit salad based on the permitted types of fruit

DRINKS

- Water, spray water, or flavored water is a great choice.
- Tea: black tea, white and green tea, fruit tea of the permitted types of fruit, Chai tea, dandelion tea, peppermint tea, rooibos tea, rosehip tea. Do not leave the tea for too long and drink in reasonable quantities.

- Alcohol is best to limit.
- Soft drinks.
- Drink decaffeinated coffee.

With proper preparation, you can still enjoy the holidays!

The 3 diet phases:
1. The Elimination Diet. This phase lasts approximately four weeks, during which you remove all high FODMAP foods from your diet. After 4 weeks, the evaluation of your symptoms will take place. Has it improved? If not, the diet is not the solution for you. If it gets better, continue with:
2. The introduction phase. Here you add certain products from the FODMAP groups to your diet, and you keep track of the symptoms that you experience. In the end you have a list of products that you can and cannot eat. Once you have established that, you are in:
3. The FODMAP way of life. This is the final phase of the diet. You know the products you are sensitive to, and you avoid them. All other FODMAPs are included in your diet. This last part is essential! Because it is not good to stay within the elimination phase for a more extended period. Elimination diets are usually very restrictive, and it is challenging to meet your nutrient and fiber needs. A shortage of nutrients or fiber is not suitable for your health. So please do not stay in the elimination phase!

In the FODMAP way of life, it is essential to retest yourself for your food sensitivities approximately every six months. Your gut renews itself every three days, and your gut bacteria and gut health are continually changing. It may be that a food hypersensitivity that you now have will no longer be present in 3 months. It would be a shame if you never tested again and never discovered that you could eat certain foods again!

Low And High Fodmap Products

These lists are ideal for providing insight into the products that you can and cannot eat.

- It is not always clear who made a list, is it a reliable source?

- Usually, the lists are quite old, when was it last updated?

- It is not easy to find a specific product in a list written/printed on paper.

The Best List Of Fodmap Products

It is recommended to use the Low FODMAP Diet app available on Android and Apple. This app is updated when the university has tested a new product and gives you information about low FODMAP products and checking portion sizes. This way, you always have a reliable source of information about FODMAP in your pocket.

The app uses a traffic light system.

Green products are the ones that you can eat unlimited.

Orange products can be used per 1 product per meal in the stated quantities.

Red products must be avoided altogether.

This approach helps you choose the products that suit you.

High fodmap products

Consider a sample list of products in the high FODMAP carbohydrate groups.

Vegetables and beans

- garlic;
- onion;
- artichoke;
- asparagus;

- fresh beets;
- black Eyed Peas;
- Beans
- cauliflower;
- celery root;
- falafel
- sauerkraut (e.g. sour);
- beans;
- leek;
- mushrooms;
- peas;
- pickled vegetables;
- savoy cabbage;
- soya beans;
- green onions;
- Shallot.

Fruits
- apples
- apricots
- avocado;
- bananas, ripe;
- blackberry;
- sweet cherry;
- dates;
- feijoa;
- figs;
- grapefruit;
- guava;
- mango;
- nectarines;
- peaches;
- pears
- persimmon;

- dried pineapple;
- plums
- Garnet;
- prunes
- raisins;
- sea buckthorn;
- canned fruits;
- Watermelon.

Meat

- sausages;
- Chorizo.

Cereals, bread, cookies, pasta, nuts and cakes

Products containing wheat, such as:

- cookies, including chocolate;
- wheat bread;
- breadcrumbs;
- Cakes
- wheat-based cereal bar;
- croissants
- donuts
- egg noodles;
- Cupcakes
- cakes
- pasta, wheat more than 1/2 cup, cooked;
- wheat bran;
- wheat cereals;
- Wheat flour;
- wheat germ;
- wheat noodles;
- Wheat rolls.

Bread:

- grain;

- oat;
- from pumpkin;
- almond flour;
- amaranth flour;
- barley, including flour;
- cereal bran;
- couscous;
- granola;
- cereal muesli;
- pistachios;
- rye crackers;
- Semolina.

Seasonings, sauces, sweets, sweeteners and spreads
- agave;
- fructose;
- sauce if it contains onions;
- corn syrup;
- Hummus
- honey;
- jam;
- strawberry jam;
- molasses;
- pesto;
- quince paste;
- candy without sugar;
- tahini pasta

Sweeteners and the corresponding E number:
- inulin;
- isomalt (E953 / 953);
- lactitol (E966 / 966);
- maltitol (E965 / 965);
- mannitol (E241 / 421);
- sorbitol (E420 / 420);

- xylitol (E967 / 967).

Prebiotic products

The following substances can be hidden in yoghurts, bars and snacks:

- FOS - fructooligosaccharides;
- inulin;
- oligofructose.

Beverages and Protein Powders

- fruit and herbal teas with apples, chamomile, fennel, dandelion;
- large quantities of fruit juices
- chocolate flavored malt drink;
- meal replacement drinks containing milk-based products;
- high fructose corn syrup (HFCS) soda;
- Sports drinks.

Milk products

Milk:

- Cow
- goat;
- condensed;
- sheep;
- sour cream;
- yogurt;
- kefir;
- buttermilk;
- cheese, cream;
- ricotta
- custard;
- ice cream;

Low FODMAP Product List

A low FODMAP diet can be complicated, but this list of healthy foods makes dieting a lot easier.

Vegetables and Beans
- alfalfa;
- bean sprouts;
- canned and pickled beets;
- black beans - 45 gr;
- Bok Choi;
- broccoli , total - 1/2 cup;
- Brussels sprouts - 2 sprouts;
- zucchini;
- ordinary and red cabbage to 1 cup;
- carrot;
- petiole celery - 20 gr;
- chicory leaves;
- chickpeas - 1/4 cup;
- chilli;
- corn - only in small quantities - 1/2 ear;
- zucchini ;
- cucumber;
- eggplant;
- dill;
- Green pepper;
- ginger;
- leek leaves;
- lentils - in small quantities;

Salad:
- iceberg;
- radicchio;
- romaine;
- olives;
- parsnip;
- peas - 5 pods;
- pickled gherkins;
- potatoes;

- pumpkin;
- radish;
- green onions;
- seaweed / nori;
- chard;
- spinach;
- sun-dried tomatoes - 4 pcs;
- swede;
- tomato - canned, cherry, ordinary;
- Turnip.

Fruits
- unripe bananas;
- Blueberries
- cranberries - 1 tbsp. l.;
- pitahaya;
- lingonberry;
- grapes;
- guava, ripe;
- melon;
- kiwi;
- lemon, including lemon juice;
- lime, including lime juice;
- mandarin;
- orange;
- passion fruit;
- papaya;
- a pineapple;
- raspberry;
- rhubarb;
- Strawberry.

Meat, poultry and meat substitutes
- beef;
- chicken;

- kangaroo;
- lamb;
- pork;
- prosciutto;
- Ham and turkey breast.

Fish and seafood

- canned tuna;
- fresh fish, for example:
- cod;
- haddock;
- flounder;
- salmon;
- trout;
- Tuna.

Seafood:

- crab;
- lobster;
- mollusks;
- oysters
- Shrimp.

Cereals, bread, cookies, pasta, nuts and cakes

Gluten Free Bread:

- corn;
- oat;
- rice;
- almonds - maximum 15;
- shortbread cookies - only 1;
- Brazilian nut;
- Bulgur - 1/4 cup boiled, portion 44 g;
- buckwheat;
- buckwheat flour;
- corn flour;

- corn flakes - 1/2 cup;
- coconut - milk, cream, pulp;
- corn tortillas, 3 tortillas;
- hazelnuts - maximum 15;
- macadamia nuts;
- millet;
- oatmeal, 1/2 cup;
- peanut;
- pecan - maximum 15;
- pine nuts - a maximum of 15;
- polenta;
- popcorn;
- cereals and oatmeal;
- potato flour;
- pretzels;
- pasta - up to 1/2 cup;
- rice:
- Basmati
- brown;
- rice noodles;
- white;
- rice flour;

Seeds:
- chia;
- hemp;
- poppy seeds;
- Pumpkins
- sesame seeds;
- sunflower;
- Walnuts.

Seasonings, sauces, sweets, sweeteners and spreads
- aspartame;
- acesulfame K;

- almond oil;
- capers in vinegar;
- salted capers;

Chocolate:

- dark;
- milk - 3 squares;
- white - 3 squares;
- Dijon mustard;
- erythritol (E968 / 968);
- fish sauce;
- golden syrup;
- glucose;
- glycerin (E422 / 422);
- strawberry jam / jelly;
- maple syrup;
- confiture;
- miso paste;
- pesto sauce - less than 1 tbsp. l .;
- peanut butter;
- rice malt syrup;
- saccharin;
- hot chili sauce - 1 tsp;
- stevia;
- sucralose;
- sugar - also called sucrose;
- tomato sauce - 2 bags, 13 gr;
- vinegar;
- Apple cider vinegar - 2 tbsp. L.;
- Balsamic vinegar - 2 tbsp. l.;
- rice wine vinegar;
- vasaabi;
- Worcestershire sauce.

Beverages and Protein Powders

Alcohol is an irritant for the intestines, limited intake is recommended:

- beer - 1 bottle;
- vodka;
- gin;
- whiskey;
- wine - 1 glass;
- coffee;
- kvass;
- lemonade - in small quantities;

Protein powders:

- egg white;
- pea protein - up to 20 gr;
- rice protein;
- whey protein isolate;

Soft drinks - such as diet cola, in small quantities, since aspartame and acesulfame K can be irritants;

- tea:
- the black;
- green;
- mint;
- white;
- Water.

Dairy and Eggs

- butter;
- cheese:
- brie;
- Camembert;
- Cheddar;
- feta;
- Mozzarella;
- Parmesan;

- ricotta - 2 tablespoons;
- Swiss;
- eggs
- milk:
- almond;
- hemp;
- milk without lactose;
- macadamia;
- oatmeal - 30 ml;
- rice - up to 200 ml;
- sorbet;

Menu for the week: 7 days Fodmap Diet Plan

A 7-day low FODMAP diet plan is a diet plan that helps you temporarily exclude FODMAPs from your diet, which is a proven trigger for irritable bowel syndrome.

Day 1

Breakfast

A cocktail of unripe banana, frozen strawberries, flax seeds and almond milk, green tea.

Lunch

Baked salmon + low FODMAP vegetables + 1 cup cooked brown rice (for fiber).

Dinner

Fresh spring salad. Choose a maximum of 3 vegetables (from the list), add protein, if desired, and green onions.

Day 2

Breakfast

1/2 cup oatmeal + water or lactose-free milk, topped with ½ green banana.

Lunch

Brown Rice Noodles and Shrimp Vegetarian Roast

Dinner

Pumpkin and Carrot Risotto

Day 3

Breakfast

Oatmeal with Green Banana and Chocolate

Lunch

Quinoa with chicken leg and parmesan + low FODMAP vegetables and canned tomatoes

Dinner

Salad of lettuce, bell pepper, tomato, alfalfa sprouts, seasoned with sauce, a cup of weak black tea.

Day 4

Breakfast

Black coffee, 2 whole eggs and ½ cup oats

Lunch

Baked chicken with green onions, sunflower oil, salt, pepper, brown rice.

Dinner

Romaine salad with 120 gr grilled chicken and chopped hard-boiled egg with olive oil dressing

Day 5

Breakfast

Black coffee, 3 whole eggs and 85 grams of ham

Lunch

170 grams of fried tuna with eggplant and mint tea

Dinner

½ cup steamed brown rice, 120 gr grilled chicken with coleslaw

Day 6

Breakfast

60 g hard cheese, 2 whole eggs, 1 slice of gluten-free bread (toasted)

Lunch

Braised beef with parsnip.

Dinner

170 gr grilled pork chop with vegetable salad and vinegar dressing.

Day 7

Breakfast

Omelet with cheddar cheese, bell pepper, spinach, olives and tomatoes, gluten free toast, coffee

Lunch

Sandwich with gluten-free bread, turkey, Swiss cheese, alfalfa sprouts, a glass of lemonade.

Dinner

170 gr baked cod and fried bell pepper.

Here are examples of fodmap recipes

If a person suffers from symptoms of food intolerance, then a low-calorie diet is the only proven method to determine which foods cause these symptoms.

Below are some low-FODMAP recipes to help you get started.

Lettuce Tacos With Chicken To The Shepherd

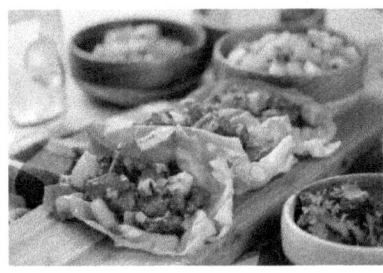

Preparation time: 1 h 20 minutes

Cooking time: 35 minutes

Ingredients

- 6 Servings
- 50 grams of achiote for the marinade
- 1/4 cup of apple vinegar for the marinade
- 3 pieces of guajillo chile clean, deveined and seedless, hydrated for the marinade
- 2 pieces of wide chili clean, deveined and seedless, hydrated for the marinade
- 3 garlic cloves for the marinade
- 1/4 piece of white onion for the marinade
- 1/2 cup pineapple juice for marinade

- 1 tablespoon salt marinade
- 1 tablespoon fat pepper for marinade
- 2 pieces of clove for the marinade
- 1 tablespoon oregano for the marinade
- 1 piece of roasted guaje tomato, for the marinade
- 1 tablespoon cumin for the marinade
- 1 piece of boneless and skinless chicken breast, cut into small cubes
- 1 tablespoon of olive or flax oil
- Enough of French Lettuce Eva
- 1/2 piece of pineapple cut into half moons
- 1/2 cup chopped coriander
- 1/2 cup finely chopped purple onion
- To the taste of tree chili sauce to accompany
- To the taste of lemon to accompany

Preparation

1. For the marinade, blend the achiote, vinegar, chilies, garlic, onion, juice, salt, pepper, cloves, oregano, tomato, and cumin until a homogeneous mixture is obtained.
2. Put the chicken and the marinade inside a bowl with the shepherd marinade for 1 hour in refrigeration.
3. Heat a pan over medium heat with the oil and cook the chicken you marinated until it is cooked. Reserve covered.
4. Heat a grill over high heat, roast the pineapple until golden brown, remove and cut into cubes, reserve.
5. On a table place sheets of French Lettuce Eva®, add the chicken to the shepherd and serve with the roasted pineapple, cilantro, onion, served with a little sauce and lemons.

Nutritional information

- Percentage of daily values based on a 2,000-calorie diet.
- Calories   92.2   kcal 4.6%
- Carbohydrates   22.3   g 7.4%
- Proteins   1.6   g 3.2%

- Lipids   0.9   g 1.3%
- Dietary fiber   2.9   g 5.8%
- Sugars   6.6   g 7.4%
- Cholesterol   0.0   mg 0.0%

Apple Salad With Garbanzo And Nut

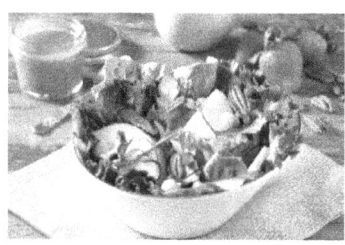

Preparation time: 10 minutes

Cooking time: 2 min

Ingredients

1 Portion

- 2 cups chopped Eva Lettuce
- 1 cup chopped arugula
- 1 cup of green apple cut into thin slices
- 1/4 cup of toasted chickpea
- 1/4 cup of toasted walnut
- 2 teaspoons of olive oil
- 1/4 cup strawberry
- 1 pinch of salt
- 1 pinch of pepper
- 3 tablespoons of raspberry vinegar

Preparation

1. In a bowl add the lettuce, the arugula, add the green apple, with the chickpea and the walnut. Mix perfectly well. Reservation.
2. Add the olive oil with the strawberry, salt, pepper and raspberry vinegar to the blender. Blends perfectly well.
3. Serve the salad on a plate and add the strawberry vinaigrette to garnish.

    Enjoy

Nutritional information

Percentage of daily values based on a 2,000-calorie diet.

- Calories   878   kcal 44%
- Carbohydrates   122   g 41%
- Proteins   36.2   g 72%
- Lipids   34.1   g 52%
- Dietary fiber   36.5   g 73%
- Sugars   50.3   g 56%
- Cholesterol   0.0   mg 0.0%

Sheet Pan Steak Fajitas

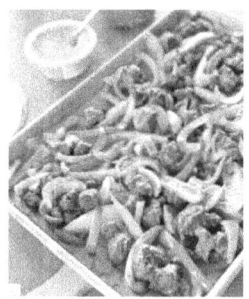

Ingredients:

- 2 teaspoons chili powder
- 2 teaspoons ground cumin
- 1 teaspoon smoked paprika
- Salt and black pepper, to taste
- 1 1/2 pounds, sirloin steak, cut into thin strips
- 1 green bell pepper, cut into strips
- 1 orange bell pepper, cut into strips
- 1 red onion, cut into wedges
- 4 to 5 cloves garlic, minced
- 3 tablespoons olive oil
- 2 tablespoons freshly squeezed lime juice
- 6 (8-inch) flour, corn tortillas or carb balance, warmed

Preparation:

1. Preheat oven to 425 degrees F. Lightly oil a baking sheet or coat with nonstick spray.
2. In a small bowl, combine chili powder, cumin, paprika, 2 teaspoons salt and 2 teaspoons pepper.
3. Place steak, bell peppers, onion and garlic in a single layer onto the prepared baking sheet. Stir in olive oil and chili powder mixture; gently toss to combine.

4. Place into oven and bake for 25 minutes, or until the steak is completely cooked through and the vegetables are crisp-tender. Stir in lime juice.
5. Serve immediately with tortillas.

Love Sheet Pan Dinners? Check out these meals! Sheet Pan Tuscan Chicken, Sheet Pan Egg in the Hole, Breaded Pork Chop Sheet Pan Dinner, and One Pan Balsamic Chicken.

Shopping lists:

- 2 teaspoons chili powder
- 2 teaspoons ground cumin
- 1 teaspoon smoked paprika
- Salt and black pepper
- 1 1/2 pounds, sirloin steak
- 1 green bell pepper
- 1 orange bell pepper
- 1 red onion
- 4 to 5 cloves garlic
- 3 tablespoons olive oil
- 2 tablespoons freshly squeezed lime juice
- 6 (8-inch) flour, corn tortillas or carb balance

Nutrition Fact:

- Calories 440Calories from Fat 297 % Daily Value
- Fat 33g 51%
- Carbohydrates 5g 2%
- Fiber 1g 4%
- Sugar 1g 1%
- Protein 31g6 2%
- Vitamin C 78.4mg 95%
- Iron 3.7mg 21%

Sheet Pan Tuscan Chicken

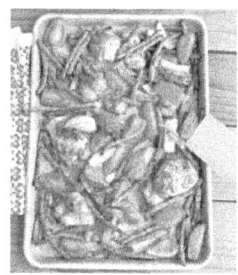

Ingredients

- 4 whole Boneless, Chicken Thighs
- 6 whole Roma Tomatoes, quartered
- 1 pound Green Beans
- 1 onion, cut into chunks
- 1 cup Olive Oil
- 1/3 cup Balsamic Vinegar
- 5 cloves Garlic, Minced
- 1 teaspoon Dried Parsley Flakes
- 1 teaspoon Salt
- 1 teaspoon Black Pepper
- 2 Tablespoons Parsley

Preparation:

1. To a bowl or pitcher, add the olive oil and balsamic vinegar, along with the garlic, parsley, salt, and pepper. Whisk it until it's well blended.
2. Place the chicken in a large zipper bag and pour in half the dressing. Seal the bag and set it aside.
3. Cut the tomatoes in quarters. Cut onion into chunks. Trim the ends off the green beans, and place the veggies in a large zipper bag. Pour in the rest of the dressing, then seal the bag and set them aside.

4. Preheat the oven to 425 degrees. Arrange the chicken and veggies on a sheet pan, Pour a little of the marinade on top of the chicken. Roast in the oven for 25 minutes, shaking the pan once during that time.

Variations

- With a few minutes left of cook time, lay slices of fresh mozzarella on each chicken breast. Return them to the oven until melted.

- Sprinkle ½ cup shredded Parmesan all over the pan as soon as you remove it from the oven. Let it sit a few minutes before serving.

Shopping lists:

- 4 whole Boneless, Chicken Thighs
- 6 whole Roma Tomatoes, quartered
- 1 pound Green Beans
- 1 onion, cut into chunks
- 1 cup Olive Oil
- 1/3 cup Balsamic Vinegar
- 5 cloves Garlic, Minced
- 1 teaspoon Dried Parsley Flakes
- 1 teaspoon Salt
- 1 teaspoon Black Pepper
- 2 Tablespoons Parsley

Nutrition Fact:

- Calories 441 Calories from Fat 198
    % Daily Value
- Fat 22g 34%
- Saturated Fat 5g 31%
- Cholesterol 119mg 40%
- Sodium 986mg 43%
- Potassium 1044mg 30%
- Carbohydrates 15g 5%
- Fiber 3g 13%

- Sugar 8g 9%
- Protein 43g 86%
- Vitamin A 1500IU 30%
- Vitamin C 26.1mg 32%
- Calcium 215mg 22%
- Iron 2.7mg   15%

Breaded Pork Chop Sheet Pan Dinner

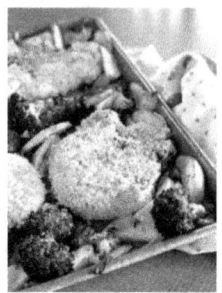

Ingredients:

- 4 (8-ounce) pork chops, bone-in, 3/4-inch to 1-inch thick
- Salt and freshly black pepper, to taste
- 2 large eggs, beaten
- 1/4 cup milk
- 1 1/2 cups Panko
- 1 Tablespoon garlic powder
- 2 teaspoons onion powder
- 1 teaspoon dried oregano
- 1 teaspoon dried parsley
- 1 teaspoon smoked paprika
- 1/4 cup vegetable oil

For The Broccoli and Apples

- 1 pound broccoli, chopped
- 1 green apple, cut into 1/2-inch wedges
- 1/2 purple onion, diced
- 3 tablespoons olive oil
- 3 tablespoon brown sugar
- 1 teaspoon dried rosemary
- Salt and black pepper, to taste

Preparation:

1. Preheat oven to 425 degrees F. Lightly oil a baking sheet or coat with nonstick spray.
2. In a large bowl, combine broccoli, onion, apple, olive oil, brown sugar, and rosemary; season with salt and pepper, to taste; set aside.
3. Season pork chops with salt and pepper, to taste.
4. In a large bowl, whisk together eggs and milk. In another large bowl, combine Panko, garlic powder, onion powder, oregano, parsley, paprika and vegetable oil; season with salt and pepper, to taste.
5. Working one at a time, dip pork chops into the egg mixture, then dredge in the Panko mixture, pressing to coat.
6. Place pork chops onto the prepared baking sheet; place broccoli mixture around pork chops.
7. Place into oven and bake for 10-12 minutes. Turn pork chops over, and bake for an additional 10-12 minutes, or until the pork is completely cooked through. Serve immediately.

Shopping lists
- 4 (8-ounce) pork chops, bone-in, 3/4-inch to 1-inch thick
- Salt and freshly black pepper
- 2 large eggs
- 1/4 cup milk
- 1 1/2 cups Panko
- 1 Tablespoon garlic powder
- 2 teaspoons onion powder
- 1 teaspoon dried oregano
- 1 teaspoon dried parsley
- 1 teaspoon smoked paprika
- 1/4 cup vegetable oil

For The Broccoli and Apples
- 1 pound broccoli, chopped
- 1 green apple, cut into 1/2-inch wedges
- 1/2 purple onion, diced
- 3 tablespoons olive oil

- 3 tablespoon brown sugar
- 1 teaspoon dried rosemary
    - Salt and black pepper, to taste

Nutrition Fact:

- Calories 471.1
- Total Fat17.0 g
- Saturated Fat5.1 g
- Polyunsaturated Fat1.6 g
- Monounsaturated Fat7.6 g
- Cholesterol212.2 mg
- Sodium165.6 mg
- Potassium899.8 mg
- Total Carbohydrate15.7 g
- Dietary Fiber1.9 g
- Sugars0.7 g
- Protein59.3 g

Eggplant Stuffed With Tomato With Tzatziki

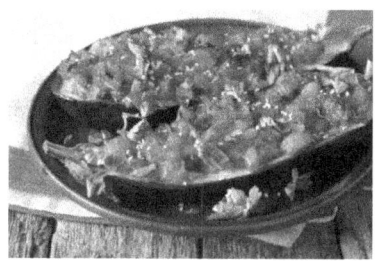

Preparation time: 10 minutes

Cooking time: 20 minutes

Ingredients 4 Portions

- 2 pieces of medium aubergine, cut in half, frayed
- 3 tablespoons olive oil
- 1 piece of finely chopped onion
- 3 garlic cloves finely chopped
- 1 tablespoon cinnamon powder
- 1 tablespoon ground cumin
- 1 tablespoon of tomato puree
- 4 pieces of tomato cut into medium cubes
- 1 tablespoon of agave honey
- 1 pinch of salt
- 1 pinch of pepper
- 1/4 cup of lemon juice
- 1 bunch of finely chopped parsley
- 1/2 bunch of finely chopped parsley
- 1/2 cup of soy yogurt
- 1 clove garlic
- 3 tablespoons finely chopped mint

- 1 pinch of paprika

Preparation

1. Preheat the oven to 200 ° C
2. Heat a small pot at medium heat with the oil, sauté the onion with the garlic, add the ground cinnamon, the cumin, the tomato puree, the tomato, and the agave honey, cook for 10 minutes, season to your liking.
3. In a table, aubergines are filled and stuffed with the tomato sautéed, baked in a tray for 20 minutes. Remove from the oven and reserve.
4. To form the tzatziki in a bowl mix the lemon juice, with the parsley, the cucumber, the yogurt, the garlic, the mint, and the paprika. Mix until a homogeneous mixture is formed.
5. Serve the aubergines with the Turkish sauce and serve with a bit of pita bread or unleavened bread.

Nutritional information

- Percentage of daily values based on a 2,000-calorie diet.
- Calories   60.8   kcal 3.0%
- Carbohydrates   9.7   g 3.2%
- Proteins   2.7   g 5.4%
- Lipids   2.1   g 3.2%
- Dietary fiber   3.2   g 6.4%
- Sugars   4.1   g   4.6%
- Cholesterol   4.6   mg 1.5%

Vegetable And Kale Soup

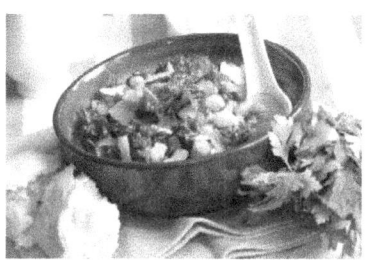

Preparation time: 10 minutes

Cooking time: 30 minutes

Ingredients

2 Servings

- 2 tablespoons of olive oil
- 1/2 piece of white onion filleted
- 1 celery stick cut in cubes
- 1 cup chopped pore
- 1 tablespoon finely chopped garlic
- 1 cup sliced mushrooms
- 1 cup mushroom filleted
- 2 cups of kale
- 1/2 piece of fennel the bulb, cut into sticks
- 6 cups of beef broth
- 1 pinch of salt
- 1 pinch of pepper
- 1/4 cup of almond

Preparation

1. Heat a medium deep pot over medium heat, add the olive oil, onion and celery until they release the aroma, add the pore, garlic and mushrooms with the mushrooms until they

start to release the juice, add the kale until I soften with the fennel. Cook for 5 more minutes.
2. Fill with the beef broth and season to your liking. Cook until it boils, covering it to prevent it from evaporating.
3. Serve in a bowl with a little fresh kale at the end and sliced almonds. Enjoy

Nutritional information

- Calories 507 kcal 25%
- Carbohydrates 65.6 g 22%
- Proteins 35.8 g 72%
- Lipids 16.3 g 25%
- Dietary fiber 11.9 g 24%
- Sugars 10.7 g 12%
- Cholesterol 0.0 mg 0.0%

Salad With Fried Goat Cheese

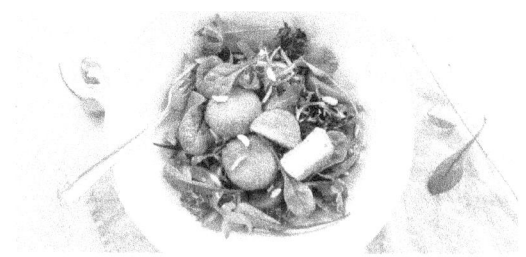

Cooking Time: 30 minutes

For 4 persons

Homemade crispy rounds of goat cheese on a bed of fresh salad with bell pepper

Ingredients

- 100 gr mixed salad
- One red pepper
- 200 gr fresh goat cheese (rounds)
- One large egg
- Oil for frying
- One tablespoon finely chopped almond
- One plate of breadcrumbs
- One plate of flour
    - Dressing
- Pepper and salt
- One tablespoon honey
- Two teaspoons lemon juice
- Three tablespoons olive oil

Preparation

1. Make sure that the goat cheese is well cold; this is the easiest way to work with it. Separate the goat cheese circles (about 12 pieces). Beat the egg on a plate. Mix the goat

cheese slices one by one through the flour, then the egg and then the breadcrumbs. And repeat the last two steps (egg and breadcrumbs) for an extra thick and crispy crust.
2. Heat the oil at 180 degrees and fry the balls for 1 minute until they are golden brown. Then drain them on kitchen paper. Separate the seeds from the bell pepper and cut into pieces and fry for 3 minutes with the olive oil in a pan.
3. Remove the pepper from the pan and pour the baking liquid into a small bowl and combine the lemon juice and honey and season with salt and pepper. Mix this dressing with the salad and add the bell pepper and serve on a plate together with the fried goat cheese. Garnish with some almond.

Nutritional information
- Calories 358.2
- Total Fat 20.7 g
- Saturated Fat 7.9 g
- Polyunsaturated Fat 3.5 g
- Monounsaturated Fat 7.9 g
- Cholesterol 35.9 mg
- Sodium 163.1 mg
- Potassium 470.6 mg
- Total Carbohydrate 33.5 g
- Dietary Fiber 4.7 g
- Sugars 21.1 g
- Protein 14.6 g

Steamed Cod

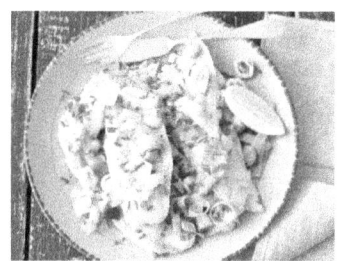

For 4 portions

Preparation: 30 min

The high-quality protein in the cod stimulates the metabolism and serves as a building material for cells, muscles, enzymes, and hormones. Valuable proteins also prevent cravings and muscle breakdown.

Ingredients

- Four cod fillets (à 150 g)
- 4 tbsps. Lemon juice
- 2 bars leek
- 3 tbsps. Rapeseed oil
- 100 ml of vegetable stock
- Salt
- Pepper
- ½ dried thyme
- ½ bunch chives (10 g)
- One organic lemon

Preparation

1. Rinse the fish fillets, pat dry and drizzle with 2 tbsps. lemon juice. Clean leeks, wash and cut into rings.

2. Heat 1 tbsps. Oil in a pan, dab fish dry, sauté for 2 minutes at medium heat. Then turn over, add the remaining lemon juice and 50 ml of vegetable stock and cover, cook for 5-7 minutes on low heat.
3. Meanwhile, heat remaining oil in a saucepan, sauté the leek rings in medium heat for 2 minutes, season with salt, pepper, and thyme. Add remaining vegetable stock and cook the leek for 5 minutes over low heat.
4. Meanwhile, wash chives, shake dry and cut into small rolls. Rinse lemon hot and cut into quarters
5. Season fish fillets and leeks with salt and pepper, arrange on plates and garnish with chives and lemon quarters.

Nutritional Fact

Calories: 226 kcal

Vegetable Lasagna

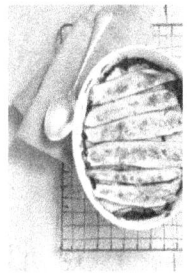

For 4 people:

Ingredients

- 80 g puy lentils
- 4 tbsp. Olive oil + a little to coat the vegetables
- 1 tomato coarse chopped beef heart
- 1 minced garlic clove
- 1 diced beetroot
- 1/2 tsp. Tamari (soy sauce)
- 1 tbsp. Dehydrated shallot dehydrated
- 1 pinch powdered cumin
- 400 g butternut squash cut into thin slices
- 300 g zucchini thinly sliced in length

Preparation:

1. Preheat the oven to temperature 170 ° c (th 5-6). Put the lentils inside a small saucepan and cover them with water. Boil it and cook for 10 to 15 minutes until al dente. Drain and reserve.
2. Meanwhile, heat the oil inside a large saucepan, then crush the tomato that will be the base of the sauce. Add garlic and beetroot, tamari, shallot, and cumin. Pour 2 tablespoons of water and cook for 15 minutes over medium heat to obtain a

thick puree. Add the lentils to the contents of the pan, add a little more water and simmer for another 5 minutes.
3. Spread half of the butternut and one-third of the zucchini in a baking dish, then cover with half of the lentil sauce. Repeat the same process and finish with a layer of zucchini. Spread them over with olive oil and cook for 45 minutes, until the vegetables are just tender.

You can replace olive oil with parsley oil.

Nutritional facts

- Calories 65
- % daily value*
- Total fat 0.2 g   0%
- Saturated fat 0 g   0%
- Polyunsaturated fat 0.1 g
- Monounsaturated fat 0 g
- Cholesterol 0 mg   0%
- Sodium 35 mg   1%
- Potassium 169 mg   4%
- Total carbohydrate 13 g   4%
- Dietary fiber 4.4 g   17%
- Sugar 3.1 g
- Protein 2.9 g   5%
- Vitamin a   85%   vitamin c   5%
- Calcium   2%   iron   4%
- Vitamin d   0%   vitamin b-6   5%
- Cobalamin   0%   magnesium   5%

Lemon-Garlic-Zucchini Salad With Walnuts And Ricotta Cheese

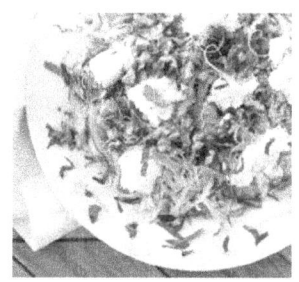

Ingredients

- Fresh basil
- Garlic
- Lemons
- Ricotta cheese
- Walnuts
- Zucchini squash
- Black pepper
- Extra virgin olive oil
- Salt

Preparation

1. Wash and dry the fresh products.
2. 2 lemons
3. 6 medium sized zucchini squash
4. Small packet of fresh basil
5. Cut off the zucchini ends. With the help of a spiralizer, the julienne peeler (or regular peeler) peels into noodle-like chopsticks. Put inside a sieve and sprinkle with salt. Place the strainer on a plate or bowl to collect excess moisture.
6. 1 teaspoon salt

7. Grate the whole shell of the lemons and sauté the lemons; transfer both into a medium bowl.
8. Peel, chop or squeeze the garlic; in a bowl and stir with oil, lemon juice and pepper.
9. Cloves of garlic
10. ⅓ cup extra virgin olive oil
11. ½ tsp black pepper
12. Put a pan over medium heat. Roughly chop walnuts. Stir the walnuts (2-4 minutes) and stir regularly.
13. ½ cup walnuts
14. Take out the basil leaves from the stems and cut into ribbons.
15. Throw the zucchini pasta with your hands and squeeze out the excess water. Do this a few times.
16. Add the zucchini into the bowl with the dressing and mix into a dressing.
17. To serve, arrange the zucchini noodles on a plate and top with ricotta cheese and walnuts and teaspoons. Sprinkle with basil and enjoy!
18. 1 (15 oz) pkg ricotta cheese

Tuna And Vegetable Salad

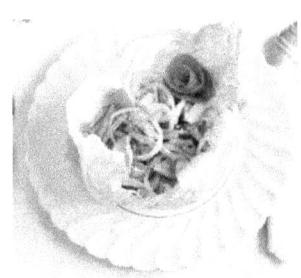

Ingredients

- 2 medium-sized zucchini (thinly cut)
- 2 medium sized carrots (cut in matches)
- 3 cans of tuna (each 5 ounces drained in water)
- 4 sticks of celery (cut and chopped)
- 1 onion (small, thinly sliced)
- 1 tablespoon of fresh, flat parsley (chopped roughly)
- 4 lettuce leaves (iceberg)
- 1/2 cup dressing (light fench)
- 2 tablespoons of yogurt
- 1 garlic clove (crushed)
- 2 teaspoons curry powder

Directions

1. Cook the zucchini and carrots in a small pan with boiling water for 1 minute. Drain and change to cold water.
2. For the dressing, put all the ingredients togetherin a small bowl and season to taste.
3. Place the zucchini and carrots with tuna, celery, onions, parsley and dressing in a medium bowl and mix gently.
4. Add the salad to the lettuce leaves and serve.

Potato And Vegetable Salad With Herb Dressing

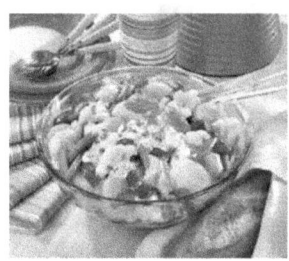

Ingredients

- 1 pound of small potatoes (peeled and halved)
- 1/2 pound of green beans (cut and cut into pieces)
- 1 cauliflower (small, cut into florets)
- 1 main salad (torn into bite-sized pieces)
- 1 red pepper (without seeds and roughly chopped)
- 1 2/3 cups of yogurt
- 3 tablespoons mayonnaise
- 2 teaspoons of basil (mince, extra leaves for garnish)
- 2 teaspoons chives (finely chopped)
- 2 teaspoons parsley (finely chopped)

Directions

1. Boil the potatoes inside boiling salted water for 15-20 minutes, until ready. Drain, cool and cut.
2. Boil beans and cauliflower florets in boiling salted water for 7-8 minutes, until soft. Drain, rinse in cold water and allow to cool completely.
3. Put the cooled potatoes with beans and cauliflower in a bowl. Add salad and pepper and mix.

4. For the dressing: put the yoghurt and mayonnaise in a bowl, add the chopped herbs, season to taste and mix freshly ground black pepper.
5. Dress over the salad, garnish with the extra basil leaves and serve.

Salad With Asparagus, Cherry Tomatoes, And Cottage Cheese

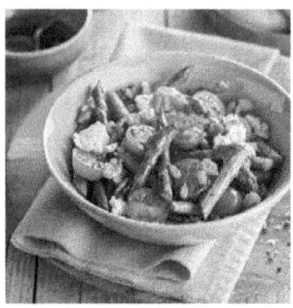

Ingredients:

- Two bunches of green asparagus
- 150 g of cherry tomatoes
- 100 g of cottage cheese
- 30 g peeled walnuts
- 30 g of kikos (toasted corn)
- 20 g of peeled sunflower seeds
- Two tablespoons of vinegar
- Four tablespoons of olive oil
- Pepper and salt

Preparation

1. Clean the asparagus. First, wash the asparagus under the stream of cold water, remove the hardest part of the stem, and cut them into pieces of the same size.
2. Put water to boil and cook. While preparing the asparagus, boil plenty of salt water in a casserole, add them and cook for 10 minutes till they are tender but whole.
3. Interrupting the cooking. Once it's done, remove them with a slotted spoon and immerse them for a few moments in a bowl of ice water to halt cooking. In this way, they will

maintain their intense green color. And then, drain them again to eliminate all the water.
4. Prepare the rest of the ingredients. Wash the tomatoes, dry them with absorbent paper and cut them in half. Drain the cottage cheese and crumble it. And cut the nuts into small pieces.
5. Make the vinaigrette. Arrange the vinegar inside a bowl. Add little salt and another pepper, and pour the oil, little by little, continuing to beat with a fork, until you get well-emulsified vinaigrette.
6. Emulator and serve. Distribute the asparagus in four bowls. Add the tomatoes, the crumbled cottage cheese, and the chopped walnuts. Dress with the previous vinaigrette. And decorate with sunflower seeds and chopped kikos.

Oven Dish With Creamy Brussels Sprouts

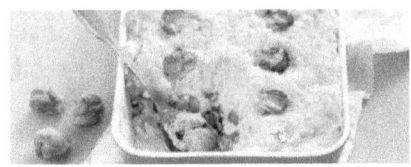

Ingredients

- 600 gr of brussels sprouts
- 250 gr bacon
- 800 gr potatoes (floury in pieces)
- 200 ml of milk
- One sweet pointed pepper
- Lump of butter
- Hand-grated cheese
- 200 gr cream cheese with herbs
- Pepper and salt
- Necessities
- Oven dish approx. 20 x 28 cm

Preparation

1. Heat the oven to 200 degrees. Boil the potatoes in approx. 15 to 20 minutes. Meanwhile, also cook the brussels sprouts for 10 minutes in a pan of water. Bake the bacon slightly crispy in a dry frying pan. Then also add the pointed bell pepper in pieces.
2. Drain the potatoes and mash them finely, add the milk, butter, pepper, and salt and mix into a puree. Add the brussels sprouts (save 5 or so for garnish) to the bacon and bell pepper. Stir in the cream cheese with herbs. Divide this mixture over a baking dish.

3. Cover with the mashed potatoes. Cut the remaining brussels sprouts in half and divide over the top of the oven dish. Sprinkle with cheese and put the oven dish in the oven for another 20 minutes.
4. Tip: for a quick variant you can also use ready-made puree.

Poké Bowl With Salmon

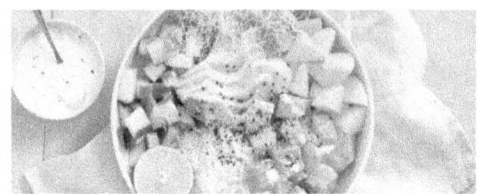

Ingredients

- 250 gr fresh salmon fillet
- One avocado
- 150 gr rice (sushi)
- Two tablespoons rice vinegar
- ½ cucumber
- Sesame seeds
- 175 g mango
- 30 g alfalfa

Sauce:

- Two tablespoons mayonnaise
- Two tablespoons lime juice
- Chili flakes to taste

Marinade salmon:

- 1 tablespoon soy sauce
- 1 tablespoon of sesame oil
- 1 tablespoon lime juice

Preparation

You can use both normal rice and sushi rice for the poke bowl. Cut the salmon into cubes, add the ingredients for the marinade and keep covered in the fridge for as long as possible. Prepare the rice and then sprinkle with rice vinegar. Cut the cucumber, mango, and avocado into pieces.

Mix the ingredients for the sauce. Divide the cubes of salmon, rice, cucumber, avocado, and mango over two bowls and divides this into separate planes. Garnish with some alfalfa, lime mayo sauce, and sesame seeds.

Burritos Of Cabbage

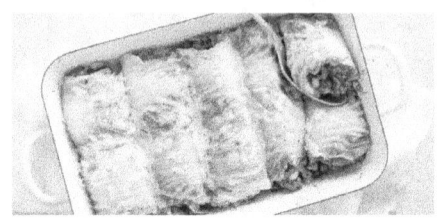

Ingredients

- One green or chinese cabbage (12 leaves)
- 300 g ground beef
- One outing
- One clove of garlic
- 400 ml diced tomatoes
- One tablespoon tomato puree
- One tablespoon of taco herbs
- One small can of corn
- Two hands of grated cheese
- 100 gr kidney beans from a sack

Requirements:

- Oven dish 26 x 18 cm

Preparation

1. Chop the onion and then garlic and fry in a pan. Add the minced meat and then the taco herbs. Bake this loose. Stir in the tomato puree and cubes and then the drained corn and kidney beans. Let this burrito filling simmer for a few minutes. Meanwhile, boil water.
2. Heat the oven to 180 degrees. Cut the cabbage leaves and boil them (per 2 or 3) for a minute or 2 in the pan and then drain well. Place two cabbage leaves next to each other so that they overlap slightly. Spoon some of the burrito filling

on one side, sprinkle with a little cheese and then carefully roll up. Don't push too hard. Repeat this with the rest of the cabbage leaves and filling. If they are all in the baking dish, sprinkle them with some extra cheese. Place the baking dish in the oven for about 15 minutes. Serve the carbohydrates with some rice (if the dish is no longer low in carbohydrates).

Waffle With Sausage Cheese Flour

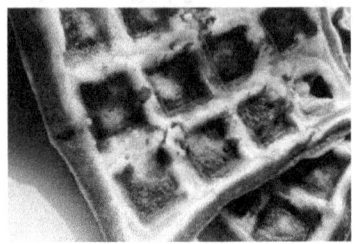

Ingredients: (for 2 waffles)

- 3 eggs
- 2 teaspoons strained yogurt
- 3 teaspoons melted butter
- 3-4 slices of sausage or bacon made at home / built in a town you trust
- 1/2 cup grater tongue cheese / or any other cheese you prefer
- 1 teaspoon old grated grated (optional)
- 1 tablespoon powdered almond (optional)

Preparation:

Warm up your waffle maker / machine. Beat the eggs, yogurt, butter. Cut your sausages into tiny pieces. Add to the mixture. Add the grated cheese and almonds if you wish and mix with a wooden spoon. Lubricate your waffle maker / machine beautifully. Share the mixture. Close the cover and do not open it for 4-5 minutes. When the time is up, lift the lid slightly and check if it is cooked. Carefully separate when cooked, serve immediately. Enjoy your meal.

Oopsie Bread

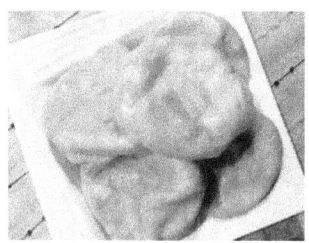

Ingredients:

- 3 eggs
- 1 teaspoon rock / himalayan salt
- 100 g homemade cream cheese (you can do by passing home-made cottage cheese and butter in the food processor)
- 1 teaspoon heaping carbonate or cream of tartar

Preparation:

Separate the yolks and the whites of the eggs. First, whisk the white together with the carbonate and salt until very solid foam. Then whisk the egg yolks until they mix well with the cream cheese. Add the solidified egg white foam on the egg yolks with the help of a wooden spoon and mix gently so that the white foams do not extinguish and the mixture does not look watery. Pour the mixture into a large tray of baking paper with the help of a ladle and the size of 6 large hamburger buns. Bake in a preheated 150 c oven until golden. Never open the oven door. When the breads are toasted, remove them from the oven, and do not remove them from the tray until they have cooled down thoroughly. Enjoy your meal!

Leek Minced Almond Flour Pastry

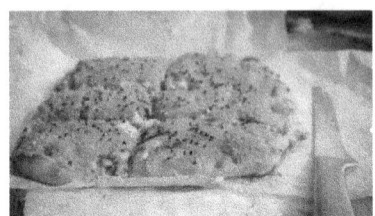

Preparation time: 30 min

Cooking time: 30 min

Service: 6 slices

This recipe is adapted from uplateanyway.com's low carb stromboli recipe.

Ingredients:
- For the dough
- 3 tablespoons kocamaar farm olive oil
- 250 gr tongue cheese
- 100 gr (1 cup + 4 tablespoons) kocamaar farm almond flour
- 1 egg (60 g)
- 1 tablespoon of apple cider vinegar
- ½ teaspoon carbonate
- ½ teaspoon of garlic or 1 small clove of garlic
- For inside
- 4-5 stalks of leek
- 2 tablespoons tomato paste
- 100 gr minced meat
- Kocamaar farm olive oil

Preparation:
1. Wash leek finely chop, mince and tomato paste and sauté in olive oil. Close the lid and leave to cook with its own juice. If necessary, add a small amount of water.

2. Grate the cheese, add 3 tablespoons of olive oil to a medium saucepan. Add the grated cheese on top and melt until it liquefies on low heat.
3. In a large bowl, mix the almond flour, eggs, carbonate, vinegar, garlic and melted cheese and turn into a dough that clings to the hand.
4. Cover a square mold of * 4-10cmx10cm * with baking paper. Wet your hands. Press the half of the dough and spread.
5. Pour the minced leek mortar over the dough. Press the remaining half on a non-stick surface to open it in a square shape and cover the mortar. Press the edges together with your fingers. Sprinkle with black seed.
6. Bake at 6-160 c for 25-30 minutes. When it is served, you can slice and serve.

Thai Pumpkin Soup

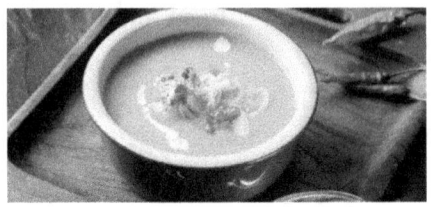

Ingredients

- 3EL Coconut Oil
- 500G Pumpkin
- 400G Carrots
- 1piece Spring Onion (50 G)
- 1piece Small Chili
- 1piece Clove Of Garlic
- 5cm Ginger (30 G)
- 1TL Turmeric
- 500ml Vegetable Stock
- 400ml Coconut Milk
- 5leaves Thai Basil
- 1piece Lime Leaf
- Prize Salt
- EL Soy Sauce
- Heap Spoon Of Coconut Oil
- Prize Black Pepper
- 1EL Lime Juice
- Fresh coriander to serve

Preparation

1. Cut off the pumpkin drink. Peel pumpkin as needed hollow out the pumpkin and weigh it. Use the same amount of carrots. Peel carrots. Cut pumpkin and carrots into large

pieces. Peel ginger and turmeric. Finely chop the spring onion, chili, ginger, turmeric, and garlic.
2. Heat coconut oil in a saucepan. Fry spring onion, ginger, chili, turmeric, and garlic. Add carrots and pumpkin and roast without browning. Add soup and coconut milk, add basil and lime leaf. Bring to a boil, add basil and lime leaf. Simmer on a flame for about 15 minutes until the vegetables are tender. Prick vegetables with a needle. If the vegetables slip off easily, it is soft.
3. Remove lime leaf and basil. Puree the soup with a hand blender.
4. Season it with soy sauce, salt, pepper, and lime juice. Serve with a little coriander.

Colorful Asparagus Caprese Salad

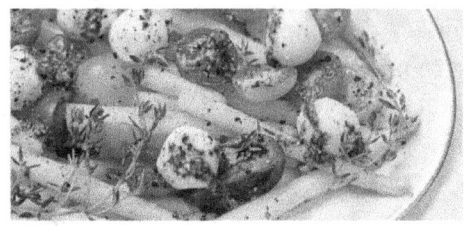

Ingredients (4 people)

- 250G tomatoes rarities
- 225G Mini mozzarella
- Topic (s) thyme
- 1.5 glasses STAUDT'S cocktail asparagus

Ingredients (4 people)

- 2TL chopped basil
- 2TL chopped parsley
- 1 Organic Lemon (Zeste & Saft)
- 1toe garlic
- 2EL olive oil
- Salt
- Pepper

Preparation

1. For the gremolata, wash the herbs, clean them, and finely chop them. Wash the organic lemon hot, rub the skin, and squeeze out the juice. Peel the garlic cloves and then chop very finely. Mix the herbs with a teaspoon of lemon zest and two teaspoons of lemon juice. Add the chopped garlic clove and the olive oil, season with salt and pepper and refrigerate in the fridge.
2. Remove the asparagus from the glasses and serve on plates. Wash, clean, and halve the tomatoes. Spread together with

the mini mozzarella on the asparagus. Drizzle with the gremolata, season with salt and pepper and garnish a few sprigs of thyme. This fits perfectly with a fresh Focaccia.

Nutritional Information

- Calories: 140.9
- Protein: 9.5 g
- Dietary Fiber: 0.5 g
- Sugars: 1.3 g

Bowl Of Shawarma

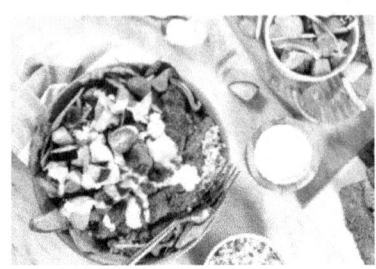

Ingredients for the shawarma

- ½ kilo of fillet or beef strips in strips
- A ¼ cup of avocado oil
- 4 cloves of garlic chopped
- 1 tablespoon garam masala
- 2 teaspoons paprika
- ½ teaspoon of sea salt
- ½ teaspoon of pepper

Ingredients for the bowl

- 4 cups of spinach and other vegetables of your choice (tomato, cucumber, broccoli)
- 2 cups of white rice
- 1 tablespoon of avocado oil
- Sea salt and pepper to taste
- A cup of cherry tomatoes and cut in half
- 1 cup cucumber chopped
- ¼ purple onion cut into thin slices
- Tzatziki sauce
- Ingredients for tzatziki sauce
- ½ cucumber peeled and finely chopped
- 1 cup of yogurt of coconut
- 2 cloves of garlic peeled cloves

- A ½ cup of fresh dill
- 1 tablespoon of lemon juice
- ½ teaspoon of salt
- ¼ teaspoon of pepper

Preparation

1. Place the sliced meat in a shallow dish. Add the avocado oil and seasonings. Cover it and put it in the refrigerator for at least 15 minutes.
2. Cook the rice while the meat is marinated. Season with salt and pepper to taste.
3. After the meat has been marinated, sauté it in a large skillet over medium-high heat until it is cooked to your liking.
4. Arm your bowls. It starts with a foundation of rice and adds your vegetable favorites.
5. To prepare the tzatziki sauce, put all the ingredients in a food processor, and mix until it has a smooth consistency. Refrigerate until used.
6. Cover with tzatziki sauce.

Nutritional Facts

- Calories: 475.0
- Protein: 41.6 g
- Dietary Fiber: 4.2 g
- Total Fat: 13.2 g

Blue Corded Chicken Breast

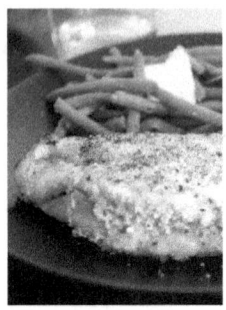

For: 4 people

Preparation time: 15 minutes

Cooking time: 10 minutes

Ingredients

- 4 chicken breasts
- 2 slices of ham
- 4 slices of Comté cheese
- 100 g of bread crumbs
- 2 eggs
- 40 g of butter
- Salt and pepper from the grinder

Preparing

Cut the chicken fillets in their thickness, leaving the 2 parts attached. Place half a slice of ham on one side. Place a good slice of county cheese and close the chicken cutlet. In a plate, beat 2 eggs with a fork to make an omelet. In another plate, pour bread crumbs. Dip the chicken breast with the ham and cheese on the plate with the eggs and dip in the bread crumbs. Bread crumbs will stick on the escape thanks to the eggs. Let the blue strips cook in the pan in the butter for 4 to 5 minutes on each side.

Nutrition Facts
- Serving Size grams (136 g)
- Serving per 1; Calories 120 cal
- Calories from Fat 0.00
- Amount per Serving % DV
- Total Fat 1.5 g 2 %
- Total Carbohydrate 0 g 0 %
- Dietary Fiber 0 g 0 %
- Sugars 0 g
- Other Carbohydrate 0.00 g
- Protein 27 g

Duck Breast With Mirabelle Plums

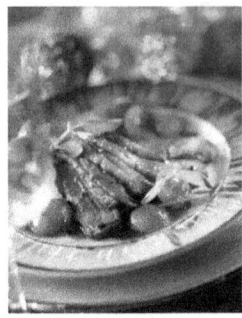

For: 4 people

Preparation time: 15 minutes

Cooking time: 15 minutes

Ingredients

- 2 duck breast (or fillet) approximately 350 g each
- 300 g frozen Mirabelle plums (or fresh)
- 1 tsp. chicken, ground coffee
- 3 cl of plum brandy
- 50 g of cold butter
- Salt and pepper from the mill

Preparation

1. Let the Mirabelle thaw at room temperature.
2. Remove some fat from the sides of the breasts. Cut the skin in crosspieces, using a sharp knife. Put them skin side in a hot pan, without adding fat. Cook for 6 minutes on high heat. Turn them over and cook for 4 minutes. Let them rest on a plate covered with aluminum foil.
3. Empty the grease from the pan without wiping it. Throw in Mirabelle plums and cook for 2 to 3 minutes while stirring. Remove them from the pan and keep them warm. Replace with the bottom of poultry diluted in water and the brandy.

Bring to the boil by peeling off the cooking juices with a wooden spoon. Stir in small pieces of butter while whisking.
4. Slice the duck breasts. Stir the juice in the sauce. Mix.
5. Arrange the slices of filleted duck on the plates, Pour the sauce and add the mirabelles. Serve immediately.

Nutrition Facts
- Calories 102(427 kJ)
- Calories from fat 32
- % Daily Value 1
- Total Fat 3.5g5%
- Sat. Fat 1.1g5%
- Cholesterol 64mg21%
  - Sodium47mg2%
- Total Carbs.0g0%
- Dietary Fiber0g0%
- Protein16.5g

Steamed Cod

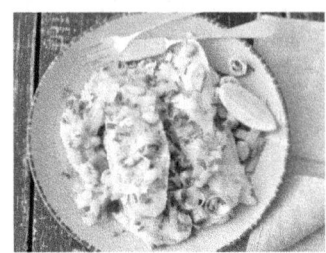

For 4 portions

Preparation: 30 min

The high-quality protein in the cod stimulates the metabolism and serves as a building material for cells, muscles, enzymes, and hormones. Valuable proteins also prevent cravings and muscle breakdown.

Ingredients

Four cod fillets (à 150 g)

4 tbsps. Lemon juice

2 bars leek

3 tbsps. Rapeseed oil

100 ml of vegetable stock

Salt

Pepper

½ dried thyme

½ bunch chives (10 g)

One organic lemon

Preparation

1. Rinse the fish fillets, pat dry and drizzle with 2 tbsps. lemon juice. Clean leeks, wash and cut into rings.

2. Heat 1 tbsps. Oil in a pan, dab fish dry, sauté for 2 minutes at medium heat. Then turn over, add the remaining lemon juice and 50 ml of vegetable stock and cover, cook for 5-7 minutes on low heat.
3. Meanwhile, heat remaining oil in a saucepan, sauté the leek rings in medium heat for 2 minutes, season with salt, pepper, and thyme. Add remaining vegetable stock and cook the leek for 5 minutes over low heat.
4. Meanwhile, wash chives, shake dry and cut into small rolls. Rinse lemon hot and cut into quarters
5. Season fish fillets and leeks with salt and pepper, arrange on plates and garnish with chives and lemon quarters.

Nutritional Fact

Calories: 226 kcal

Soup With Rice, Potatoes And Chicken

Boil 60 g of chicken with spices for 30 minutes.

Small chop 70 g of potatoes.

Then chop 1 head of onion and fry it.

Then pour potatoes and 30 g of rice into the broth, boil the composition for 15 minutes.

Salt, put bay leaf and leave to infuse for about half an hour.

Conclusion

The FODMAP limited diet is an effective treatment method for patients with irritable bowel syndrome (PDS) for whom healthy lifestyle recommendations do not provide adequate improvement of the symptoms. The FODMAP diet was developed at Monash University (Melbourne) in Australia by PR Gibson and SJ Shepherd.

The FODMAP (fermentable oligosaccharides, disaccharides, monosaccharides, and polyols) diet consists of a restriction of fermentable oligosaccharides (FOS / GOS), disaccharides (lactose), monosaccharides (fructose) and polyols (including mannitol, sorbitol). If FODMAPs are poorly resorbed in the small intestine and (partly) end up undigested in the colon, complaints can arise.

These complaints arise as a result of the rapid fermentation of FODMAPs by the colon bacteria. During this fermentation, gases are released, causing complaints such as gas formation, abdominal pain, nausea, and flatulence. Osmosis causes diarrhea.

Avoiding FODMAPs leads to complaints reduction (symptom control). Studies show that about 75% of PDS patients reduce symptoms with this diet. If a diet contains many FODMAPs, it may be considered to first limit the diet to a reasonable amount of FODMAPs, before moving on to a LOW-FODMAP diet.

It is essential that celiac disease is excluded prior to starting the diet.

The low FODMAP diet is low in gluten and thus influences the diagnosis of celiac disease.

Celiac disease can be excluded by serology; determine IgA-tTGA / EMA

In case of positive serology followed by histology MDL physician (duodenal biopsy).

Intensive involvement by the dietitian in following the FODMAP diet is essential to evaluate the course of complaints in a structured way and to look for a complete diet with maximum variation.

The FODMAP diet is a radical diet that entails (some) additional costs. The diet requires right motivation and sufficient intelligence from the patient.

The FODMAP diet is not lifelong

The FODMAP-poor diet helped in this way. Many people (including our clients) benefit from the diet. However, it is essential to know. The low FODMAP diet is not a lifelong diet. Of course, it is excellent if you have fewer intestinal complaints, and it is great that you have peace in your stomach! However, it is essential not to wait too long with the reintroduction phase of the FODMAP diet to reintroduce FODMAPs into your diet, and it is necessary to identify your personal carbohydrate triggers. Is the elimination phase going fantastic? If you have virtually no complaints anymore but are going to re-introduce foods without good success, consider the following:

Are you doing the reintroduction in the right way? Do you indeed only add foods that only contain a FODMAP? Reintroducing an apple, for example, makes no sense at the start of the reintroduction because an apple contains multiple FODMAPs (fructose and sorbitol). In terms of FODMAPs, honey or mango contains only fructose and NO other FODMAPs and are therefore suitable foods for the fructose test.

During the reintroduction phase, continue to stick to the diet that you did before the reintroduction phase. It may well be that you have more problems because you have been out to eat and perhaps have received more FODMAPs than intended, this can also influence your results. Then pick up your diet thoroughly.

It may well be that you suffer from other causes or errors in your diet. It is, therefore, best to get advice and guidance from your dietician who has experience with the FODMAP diet.

If you have reintroduced all FODMAPs, you are supervised by an experienced dietician, and you still have complaints, then there may be several problems. Consider, for example, other causes such as small intestinal bacterial overgrowth, histamine intolerance, or gluten sensitivity.

Also, carefully test all types of FODMAPs during the reintroduction. Start on the first day with a little bit different; the chances are that you will immediately get many complaints. And double the amount of day 1 on day 2. On the 3rd day you can (without complaints) add the FODMAP that you test with every meal.

It has been proven that the FODMAP diet reduces the amount of beneficial intestinal bacteria, such as bifidobacteria { Research here }. It is known that our gut bacteria play an essential role in health and disease; the scientists do not yet know what the long-term consequences will be for following the FODMAP diet for a long time. So.. don't forget to test all FODMAPs and re-introduce as many FODMAPs (especially fructans and galactans) into your diet as possible. Get to know your own limit per fodmap group! Don't be afraid to reintroduce food now or in a while. Your tolerance for foods also changes because your intestinal flora also changes and will come into balance. So do the diet well and get help from an expert dietitian. And... Listen to your body!

ps: And if you have been eating fodmap free or fodmap deficient for a while, it is advisable to take a broad spectrum of probiotics for at least 1 month to bring your intestinal flora back into balance.